# The Decorated Body

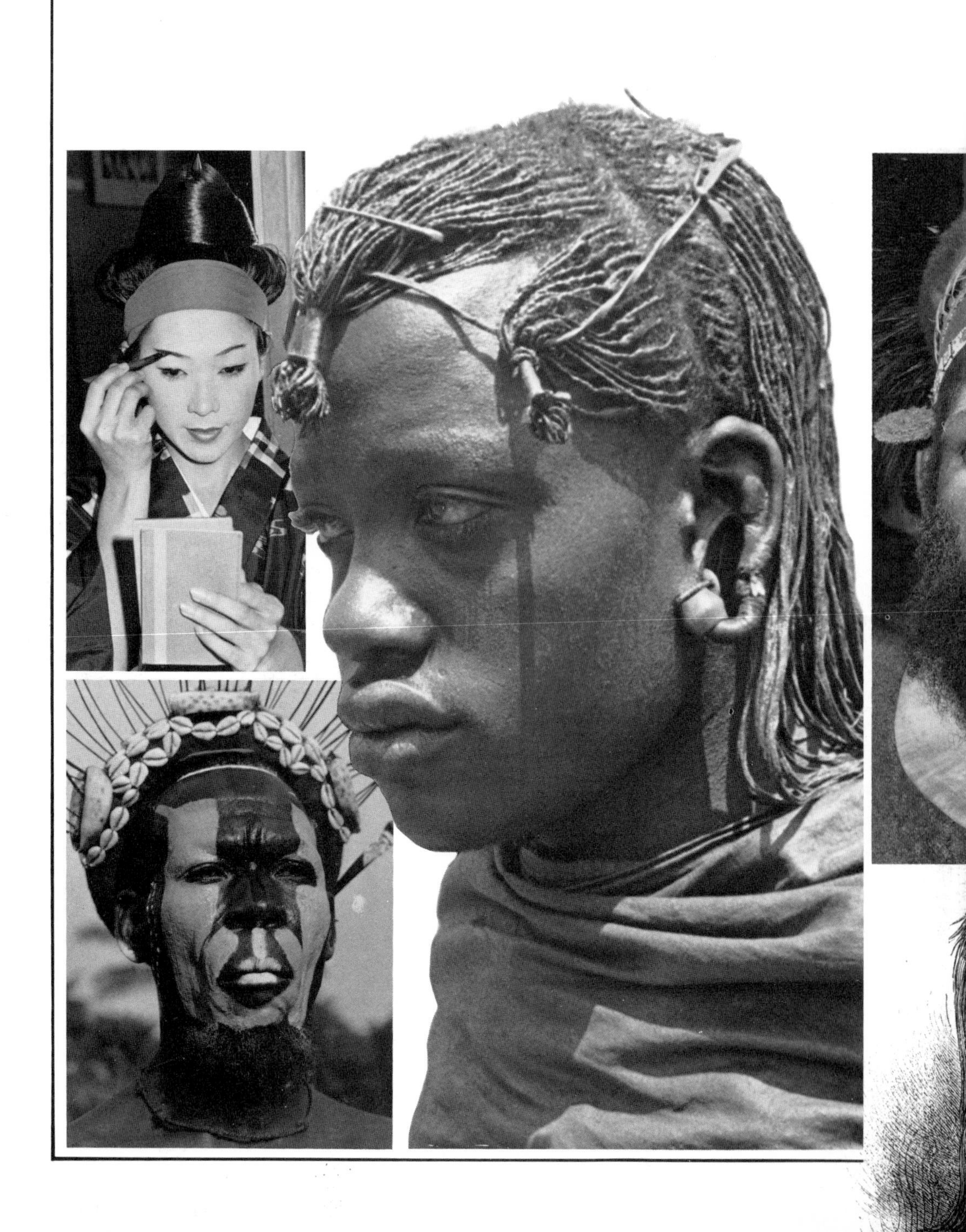

# The Decorated Body

Robert Brain

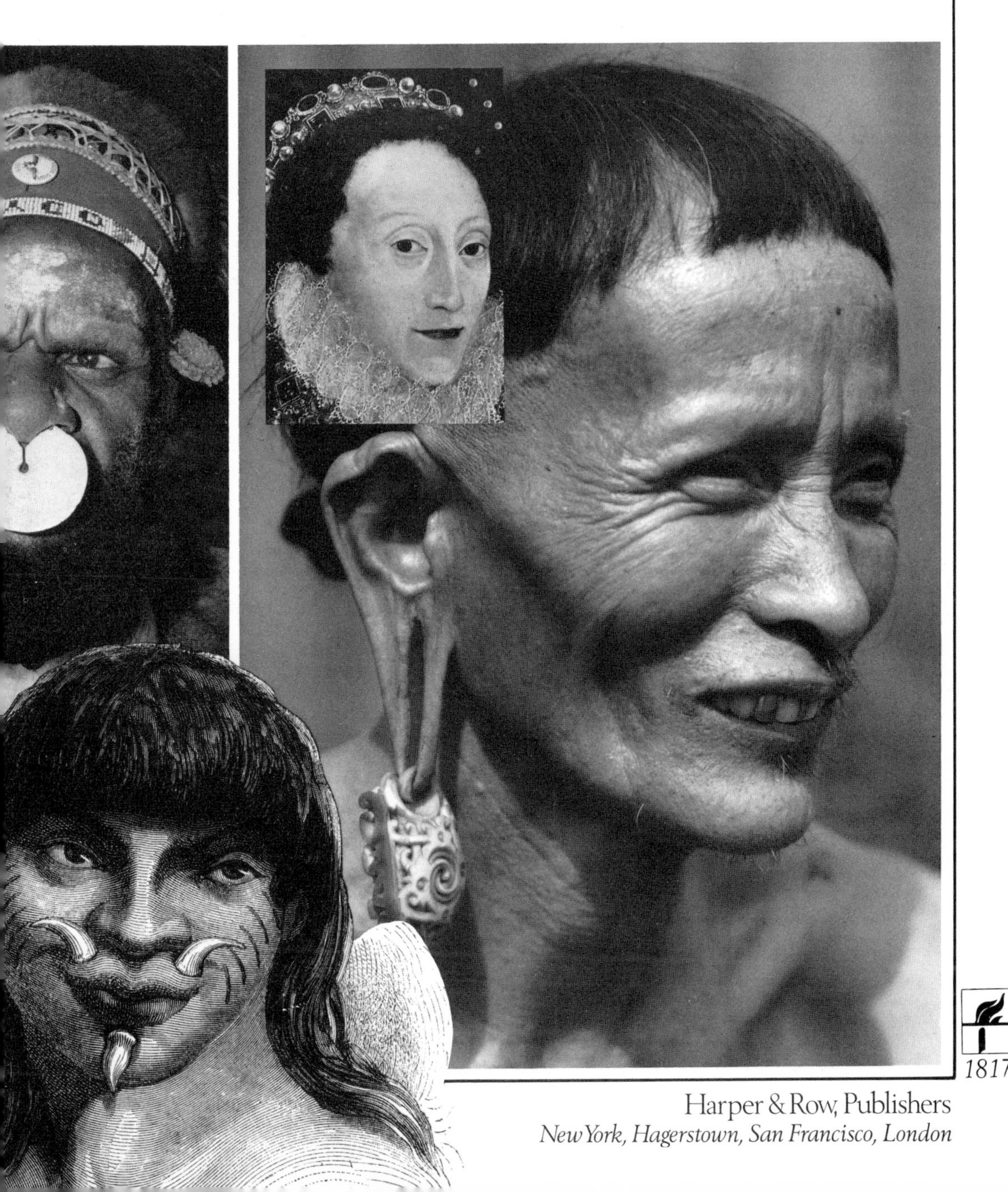

1817

Harper & Row, Publishers

*New York, Hagerstown, San Francisco, London*

**Acknowledgements**

*Title page:* (left to right, top) Camera Press × 3, Mansell Collection, Claus-Dieter Brauns; (l. to r., below) Hoa-Qui, London Editions; pp. **8/9** London Editions; **12/13** Mansell Collection; **17** J. C. Faris; **18** Granada TV (Disappearing World); **20** Lidio Cipriani; **21** (top) Australian Information Service; (bottom) Camera Press; **24/5** London Editions; **28** Moser/Tayler Collection; **29** (top) Camera Press; (bottom) Moser/Tayler Collection; **31** London Editions; **33** Andrew Strathern; **35** D. Baglin (ZEFA); **36** (top left) Robert Harding Associates; (others) J. C. Faris; **38/41** Camera Press; **49** London Editions; **53** Robert Harding Associates; (inset) Starfoto (ZEFA); **54** George & Claire Louden; **56/7** Camera Press; **59/62** London Editions; **63/5** Camera Press; **67** London Editions; **69** Ullstein-Herrnleben; **71** Bert Leidmann (ZEFA); **72** O. Luz (ZEFA); **74** (top) Alan Hutchison; (bottom & **76**) Hoa-Qui; **79** Australian Information Service; **83** Mansell Collection; **84** Camera Press; **85** and **88** (top) Mansell Collection; **88** (bottom) London Editions; **89** Mansell Collection; **91** National Gallery; **92** London Editions; **93** Mansell Collection; **95** Lidio Cipriani; **96** (top) H. W. Silvester (Rapho/Photo Researchers); (bottom) Camera Press; **98** Victoria & Albert Museum; **101** Camera Press; **103** Keystone Press Agency; **105** Camera Press; **108** Mansell Collection; **109** (left) Hoa-Qui; (right) Camera Press; **110** Mansell Collection; **116** Camera Press; **117** Mansell Collection; **118** Jack Rosen-Pix (Camera Press); **119** Mansell Collection; **123** Keystone Press Agency; **127** (top) Lidio Cipriani; (bottom) Keystone Press Agency; **129/31** V. Englebert (ZEFA); **132** Robert Harding Associates; **135** London Editions; **136/9** Camera Press; **140** London Editions; **141/4** Camera Press; **145** C. von Fürer-Haimendorf; **149** Mansell Collection; (inset) Keystone Press Agency; **150** & **151** (top) Australian Information Service; **151** (bottom) Keystone Press Agency; **152** Camera Press; **154** (top) Keystone Press Agency; (bottom) George A. Tice (Camera Press); **157** (top) Alan Hutchison; (bottom) Dr Peter W. Thiele (ZEFA); **158** (top) V. Englebert (ZEFA); (left) F. Jackson (Robert Harding Associates); (right) Claus-Dieter Brauns; **160/1** Keystone Press Agency; **165, 169** (bottom) & **171** Australian Information Service; **169** (top) & **175** John Hemming; **176** R. Smith; **179** Syndication International; **181** Camera Press. *Jacket* (front) O. Luz (ZEFA); (back) London Editions.



Published in the United States of America
by Harper & Row, Publishers, Inc., 10 East 53rd Street,
New York, New York 10022

First U. S. Edition
Library of Congress Catalog Card Number: 78-20156
ISBN 0-06-010458-9

This book was designed and produced
in the United Kingdom
by London Editions Limited,
9 Long Acre, London WC2E 9LH

Printed in England
by Balding and Mansell, Wisbech, England.

Illustrations on title page, from left to right: *top* Japanese geisha,
Masai warrior (East Africa), Hagener (New Guinea), Elizabeth I, Kelabit (Borneo);
*below* Batieke chief (Congo), South American Indian

# Contents

For Diego Calabró

# Preface

HUMAN BEINGS and human activities are complex and diverse. It is impossible either to categorize them or to generalize about them. The decoration of the body is exception. A people may be both painted and tattooed, and the motive for this may be simultaneously sexual, social and magical. The written word may in itself be too structured to describe adequately an art form which exists through man's need to express himself in visual symbols. But if a book is to be digestible it has to be organized. I have therefore divided the book into chapters, each of which deals in the main with an aspect of body decoration. Inevitably this division may at times seem arbitrary: mention of passage rites occurs in several chapters besides the one specifically devoted to it, and the same is true for the other subjects. So while I have on the whole kept to the themes in each chapter, where reason conflicted with organization I have cheerfully abandoned the latter.

*Robert Brain, Batignano, 1979*

# Introduction

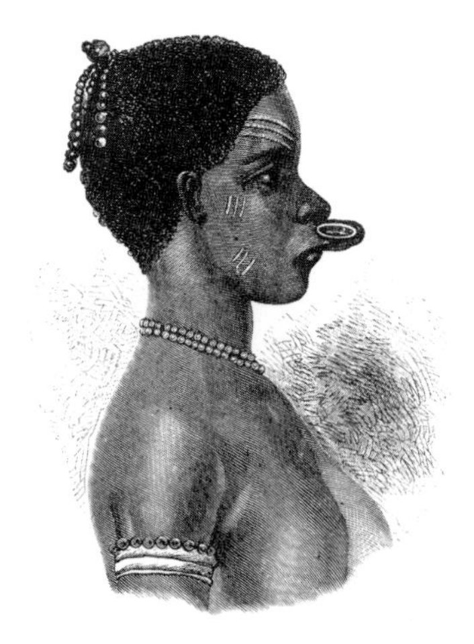

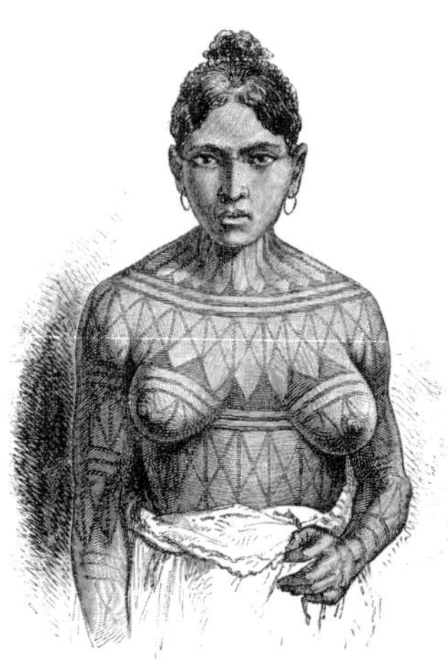

*Portraits made in the nineteenth century stressed the 'grotesque', 'wild' aspects of native people. Here,* from left to right, above and below, *are a 'Negress from the Zambesi' (from* The Races of Mankind *by Robert Brown, 1873), a 'Chief of the Marshall Islands' (from* Voyage pittoresque autour du Monde *by M. Dumont d'Urville, 1834), 'Indian, Brazil' (from* The Races of Mankind), *and an 'Australian Aborigine' (from* Voyage pittoresque). *Missionaries and administrators felt that the naked-*

IN THIS BOOK I shall attempt a cross-cultural description of the decoration of the human body, whether by tattooing, scarifying, cicatrizing, painting or otherwise changing its surface. However, I am an anthropologist, not a fashion expert or medical historian. I am concerned with earrings only if the ears are pierced, rings through the nose, not rings on the fingers, hairstyles, not hats. At the same time I shall treat body painting and body mutilation among the so-called civilized peoples on equal terms with those found among more exotic societies, for where is the divide? The Chinese lotus foot, circumcision, the tribal scar and pancake make-up are all grist to my ethnographic mill. 'Primitive' and 'civilized' cosmetics are eminently comparable. 'Cosmetics', as defined by the United States Federal Food, Drug and Cosmetic Act, is a word which can be equally applied to Melanesian, African, Polynesian and Western body art: 'articles intended to be rubbed, poured, sprinkled or sprayed on, introduced into, or otherwise applied to the human body or any part thereof for cleansing, beautifying, promoting attractiveness, or altering the appearance.'

'Primitive' and 'civilized'! I must apologize at once for the use of such shorthand terms. I use 'primitive' to refer to peoples and societies which are non-literate, small-scale, face-to-face, and associated with simple, subsistence economies. I also use 'Western' not in its strict geographical sense but to refer to those societies which in general pursue a European-cum-American way of life. And I shall be describing Western practices of body decoration as yardsticks by which we can understand 'exotic'—that is 'different'—techniques. It will soon become clear that fashionable Western techniques of make-up, plastic surgery and hair-styling differ very little from those of primitive body art, apart from the fact that the latter are more elaborately involved with ritual and social institutions.

As an anthropologist, one of my main aims is to diminish the traditional gap between the primitive and the civilized, and a comparative study of body art is as good a means as any other. Our own attitudes to the human body and its transformations have always been somewhat ambiguous; in fact, for many centuries we have declared our daubings and mutilations 'natural' and theirs 'unnatural'.

In Bernard Shaw's play *Caesar and Cleopatra* there is a passage where Caesar excuses the insular prejudices of his henchman Britannus by saying: 'He thinks the customs of his tribe and island are the laws of nature', and this has ever been the attitude of the West in general. Early travellers and missionaries, blissfully blind to their own powdered wigs and tight laces, considered all other body techniques signs of barbary and savagery.

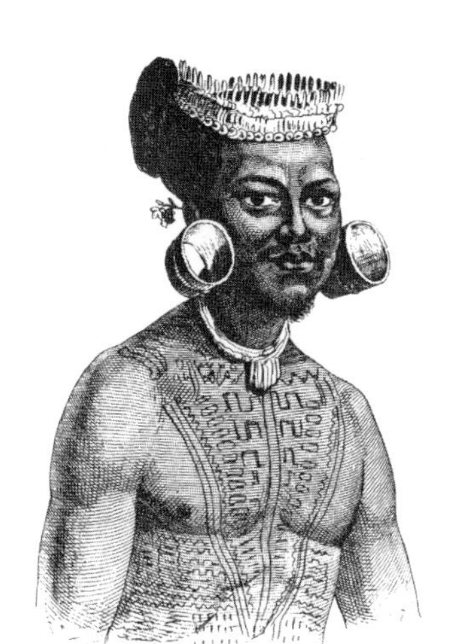

Language helps to maintain the unnatural divide. We have make-up, cosmetics, scents, creams and colorants; 'they' have twigs and swabs, animal fats and dyes. We have plastic surgery; they have mutilation. The anthropologist studying a South American Indian on a ceremonial dancing ground describes the patterns of 'coloured clay' applied with 'pork fat', and the 'ground charcoal' 'daubed' around the eyes. He might think twice about describing his wife's make-up in the same terms; yet she is most likely also wearing a red dye mixed with wax on her lips, blue, green or white pigments mixed with petroleum jelly on her eyelids, and soot and pig's fat on her brows and lashes.

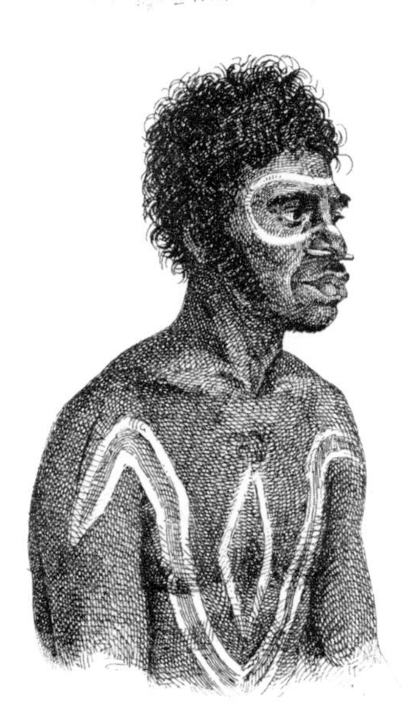

*ness of the peoples of the New World was accentuated by ornament and tattooing; they failed to understand the social significance and the symbolic statements communicated by Polynesian tattooing; and they tried to instil a feeling of guilt in the Australians towards their naked bodies. Most learned the shame of nakedness and covered their bodies with the new symbols—the clothes of Christian Western society.*

What is more savagely primitive than a fashionable woman, her bleached hair covered with tree sap? What more barbarously primitive than a queen of England who painted her breasts with artificial veins or used the fat of puppydogs mixed with apples as a hair pomade?

In the eighteenth and nineteenth centuries, when most people steadfastly refused to heed Biblical warnings to 'stay in God's image', travellers were shocked by manifestations of body decoration outside Europe and North America. In India, the English found men and women who painted their faces with sandalwood paste and musk and covered their bodies with designs of the most erotic nature. Yet in Indian religious thought a sense of bodily aesthetics was linked to an inner harmony of the soul which the pragmatic and hypocritical Englishmen could hardly grasp. In Arabia they also came across an attitude to body decoration which shocked them, since it combined the arts of seduction with religious belief. Charles Doughty described Bedouin tribesmen in 1876:

> In Arabia both men and women, townsfolk and Bedouins, where they may come by it, paint the whites of their eyes blue, with kahl or antimony; thus Mohammed Ibn Rashid

> has his bird-like eyes painted. Not only would they be more love-looking, in the eyes of the women, who have painted them and that braid their long, manly side-locks; but they hold that this sharpens too and will preserve their vision. With long hair shed in the midst and hanging down at either side in braided horns, and false eyes painted blue, the Arabian man's long head under a coloured kerchief, is in our eyes more than half-feminine; in much they resemble women.

Arabs and Hindus, however, at least had 'culture' which the Europeans with an effort could recognize as 'civilized'. When they encountered alien peoples on the American and Australian continents and in the Pacific the travellers' accounts were less polite. The intricate paintings of the South American Indians, the ritual patterns of the Australians, the splendid tattoos of the Polynesians were dismissed as 'grotesque', 'pagan', 'savage' or 'warlike'. Greenland Eskimos were described as 'sullen and untameable', more for their blue and yellow paint than for any aggressively hostile attitude—and it was much the same with the painted Picts whom the Romans found in Britain. Even Charles Darwin, who attempted to describe the Fuegians living at the tip of South America in cool scientific terms, ends up worried by the paint:

> One . . . had a fillet of white feathers tied around his head which partly confined his black coarse and entangled hair. His face was crossed by two broad transverse bars: one, painted bright red, reached from ear to ear and included the upper lip; the other, white like chalk, extended above and parallel to the first so that even his eyelids were thus coloured . . . and with their naked bodies all bedaubed with black, white and red, they looked like so many demoniacs who had been fighting . . .

A distaste for another society's art is one thing; a positive desire to eradicate it another. Travellers came and went; missionaries on the other hand usually came and stayed, and what worried them tremendously was the nakedness of their new flocks, a nakedness sometimes accentuated by paint, ornament or scarification. The missionaries and administrators, suspecting that body decoration was of greater social than cosmetic significance, communicating symbolic statements which they failed to understand, decided to expunge it.

The Tasmanians were forbidden red ochre and charcoal, grease and antimony, but they threw off the missionaries' clothes and painted their bodies again and again.

Elsewhere, the white man was more successful. The threat of the painted naked body was countered by installing a civilized sense of guilt. Armed with the story of Adam and Eve, the apple and the serpent, the native learned the shame of nakedness, covered his body with new symbols—the clothes of a Christian Western society—and ceased to 'deform' his body with tattoos, scars and greasepaint. In the Pacific, tattooing was forbidden by colonial governments and remains forbidden today. The strange thing is that missionaries and administrators accepted many compromises in their dealings with the Polynesians, the Australians and the Melanesians concerning marriage and sex, but no interdict was more severely enforced than that against tattooing. Yet Polynesian tattooing, a great art, contained no element of idolatry, no religious symbols. The missionaries saw it as pagan; the administrators as unhygienic; the philosophers described it as unnatural sado-masochism; so in the interests of pan-Christianity and Western attitudes it had to go.

What was the reason for this stubborn prejudice against the body arts? Of course we are unused to treating our bodies as a straightforward 'clay' or 'canvas' and tend to think of body art as 'disfigurement' rather than 'figuration'. Since Biblical times the painted face has been an affront to morals (in the case of women) or to our ideas of masculinity (if men paint). Jeremiah (4:30) associates paint with whores:

> And when thou art spoiled, what wilt thou do? Though thou clothest thyself with crimson, though thou deckest thee with ornaments of gold, though thou rentest thy face with painting, in vain shalt thou make thyself fair; thy lovers will despise thee . . .

Ever since, puritan attitudes have coexisted with an invincible urge to paint and transform God's work. Even the free and easy Greeks had a stern attitude to face painting. The vain Roman matron was constantly satirized: 'You'll find she has boxes with concoctions of all colours of the rainbow and you'll see the paint trickling down in warm streams on to her breast!', said Ovid, who wrote to his mistress: 'Did I not say to thee: "Cease to dye thy hair"? And now thou hast no hair to dye.' Martial wrote:

> Galla, you are but a composition of lies. Whilst you were in Rome your hair was growing on the banks of the Rhine; at night, when you lay aside your silken robes, you lay aside your teeth as well; and two thirds of your person are locked up in boxes for the night; the eyebrows with which you make such insinuating motions are the work of your slaves. Thus no man can say 'I love you', for you are not what he loves and no-one loves what you are.

Finally, Seneca writes of Thaïs:

> Cunningly wishing to exchange her disagreeable odour for some other, she, laying aside her garments, to enter the bath, cakes herself green with a depilatory or conceals herself beneath a daubing of chalk dissolved in acid or covers herself with three or four layers of rich bean-unguent. When by a thousand artifices she thinks she has succeeded in making herself safe, Thaïs still smells of Thaïs.

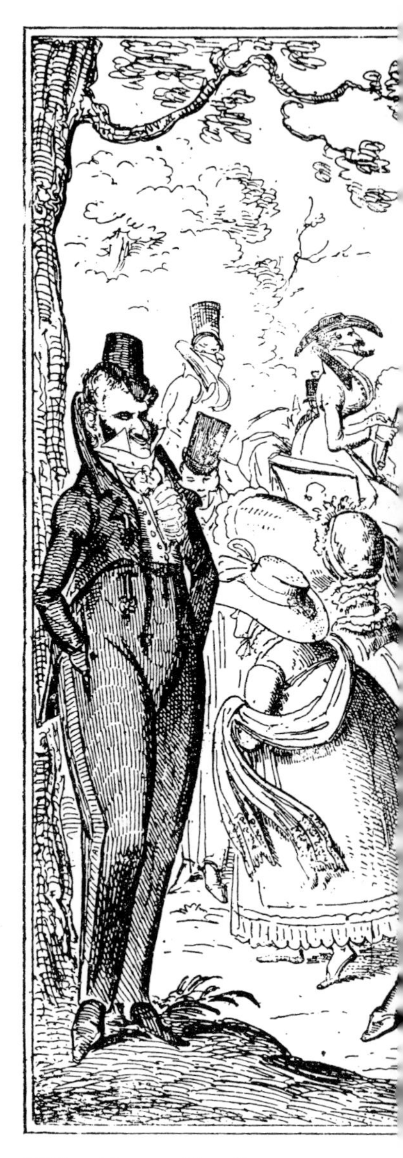

*While explorers and travellers expressed their shock at the barbarous body decoration of savages, Western sophisticates painted their faces, wore powdered wigs, and deformed their bodies through tight lacing and pointed, narrow footwear. ('Monstrosities of 1819 and 1820')*

Western cosmetics have been inextricably confused with base vanity and base sexuality. The church and its missionaries could only see body art as the influence of the devil. In England, the Puritans ranted against the extravagant cosmetics of the aristocracy and John Knox called down the wrath of God on Mary Queen of Scots as a papist and a murderess, but one has the feeling he was more incensed by her painted face than by her assassinations and religion.

Yet neither church nor parliament could stem the basic urge to transform the body. In the year of Charles I's execution a bill was introduced entitled *The vice of Painting and wearing Black Patches and Immodest Dresses of Women.* Later, an Act of Parliament designed to protect men against the false adornments of the painted, patched, plumped-out, marriage-hungry female was passed, and has never been repealed:

> All women, of whatever age, rank, profession or degree whether virgins, maids, or widows, that shall, from and after such Act, impose upon, seduce, and betray into matrimony, any of his majesty's subjects, by the scents, paints, cosmetics, washes, artificial teeth, false hair, Spanish wool, iron stays, hoops, high-heeled shoes and bolstered hips, shall incur the penalty of the law in force against witchcraft and like misdemeanours and that the marriage, upon conviction, shall stand null and void.

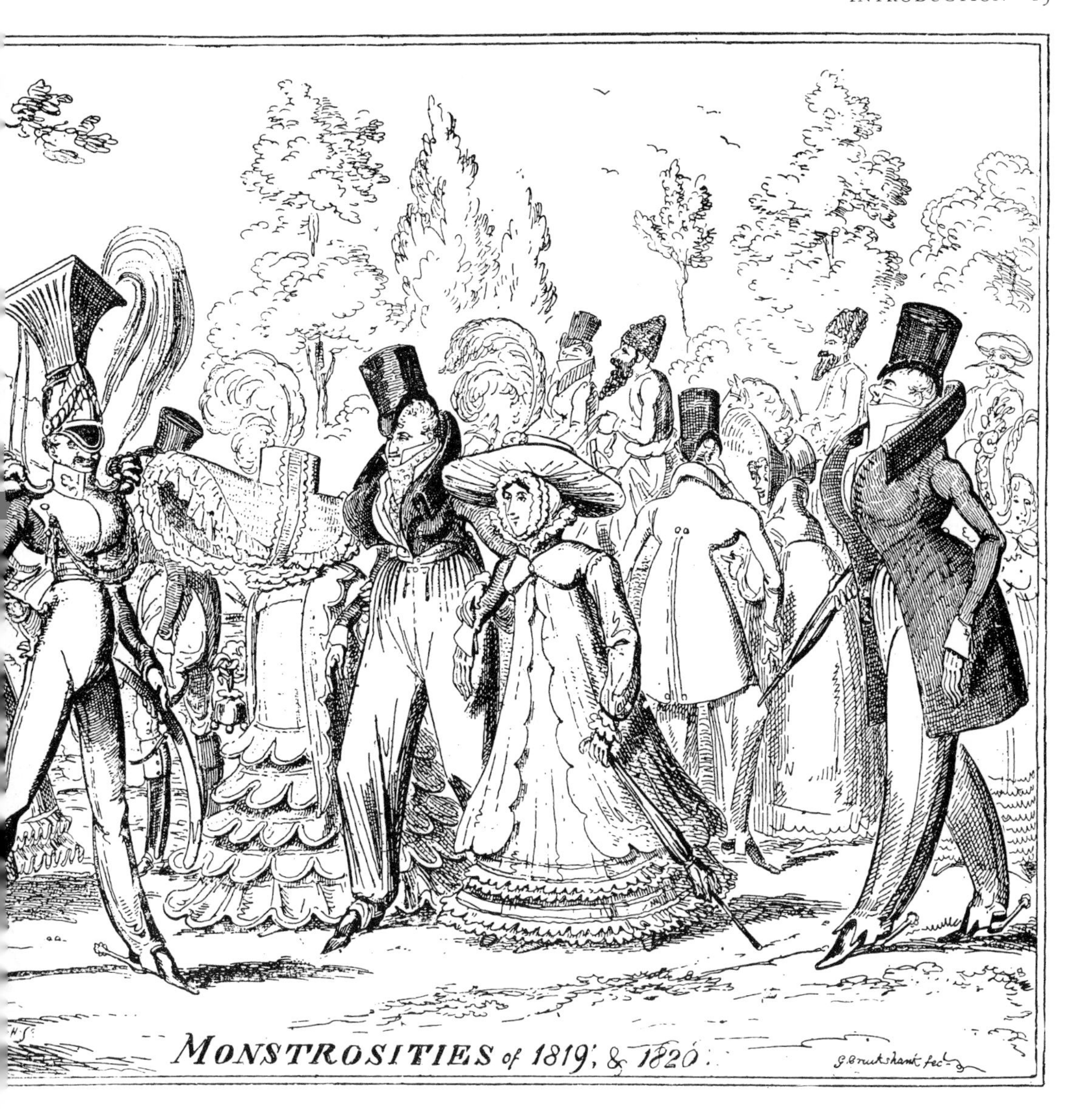
MONSTROSITIES of 1819; & 1820.
G. Cruikshank fec.

Thus throughout Western history the body arts have encountered obstacles, to put it mildly. In the mid-seventeenth century a book was devoted to the subject. Its full title is *Anthropometamorphosis; Man transform'd or the ARTIFICIAL CHANGELING. Historically Presented in the mad and cruel Gallantry, Foolish Bravery, ridiculous Beauty, Filthy Fineness, and loathesome Loveliness of most Nations, Fashioning and altering their Bodies from the mould intended by Nature with a Vindication of the Regular Beauty and Honesty of Nature, and an Appendix of the Pedigree of the English Gallant By J B (John Bulwer) 1650.*

Body decoration does seem to be a basic need which no edict from government or church can stop. The Koran and the Bible forbid body marking, yet pilgrims to Mecca and Jerusalem have always sought to tattoo their bodies as a sign of their journey. Christian pilgrims in Jerusalem were tattooed with St George, Christ on the Cross or the Virgin Mary. In Communist countries, attempts to ban cosmetics lead to the black market, and state-owned shops are forced to sell rouge and lipstick. In the West, although we spend over a billion dollars a year on cosmetics, we tend to pretend that we don't; advertisements help by implying that no deceit is involved, the purpose of the products being to liberate the 'natural' beauty within.

The irony is that having effectively killed primitive body painting, we are ourselves becoming more interested in our bodies. The stigma on cosmetic surgery is disappearing; plastic forms are available to hide or reshape the body, and there is almost no anatomical feature which cannot be made more perfect or at least more conformist. Thighs are slimmed, paunches removed, buttocks and breasts raised. Instead of secretly rouging her lips and dyeing her hair, the modern woman may indulge in wholesale body sculpture, whittling her body in the interests of fashion. Poster paints are used on the face, lashes are painted red, hair streaked with green, nails painted purple, lips mahogany. Even the yellow foundations, the spots, triangles and stripes more frequently associated with American Indians are appearing on the faces of fashion models and Punk Rock groups.

Unfortunately, Western cosmetics are imprisoned by the Western phenomenon of fashion. Paint and pattern do not celebrate in symbol the physical and social body; they celebrate the conformity of fashion. The ideal Western body is an artificial construct based on the whim of fashion. A woman of eighty may have entirely reconstructed her body half a dozen times. Before the war, a beautiful woman was a mature woman, with an emphasis on breasts and buttocks. In the 1960s and 1970s she became a wraith. The emphasis is now on youth: slim thighs and buttocks in tight jeans. In the West, if it is fashionable to be slim, all the pretty girls are slim; when the fuller figure comes they are all suddenly plump and pretty. Once, a beautiful skin was a pale, milk-and-roses complexion; then came the sun-tanned look, when the ideal body expressed idle seclusion with the bronzed appearance of youth, a look not achieved by luxurious sunny safaris or cruises but with sun-ray lamps, lotions and hair dyes.

Outside the West, the decoration of the body changes according to occasion or status. Without elaborate clothing and other devices, a whole language of body art has developed in which feelings, aesthetic sense and cultural attitudes are expressed by colourful designs, intricate tattooing, oils, fragrances and hairstyles. I shall consider non-Western body art primarily as a symbolic statement in which the decoration transmits messages about groups or individuals. By transforming the natural body into a cultural body the individual subordinates himself to the common social values of his group. The body may even become a kind of model of society, which aesthetically communicates customs and role relationships from individual to individual.

*chapter one*

# The Painted Body

*A South-eastern Nuba youth brilliantly painted with a whole body design to accentuate facial features and the form of the body. The painting stresses values associated with the young male body—physical strength, prowess, and beauty.*

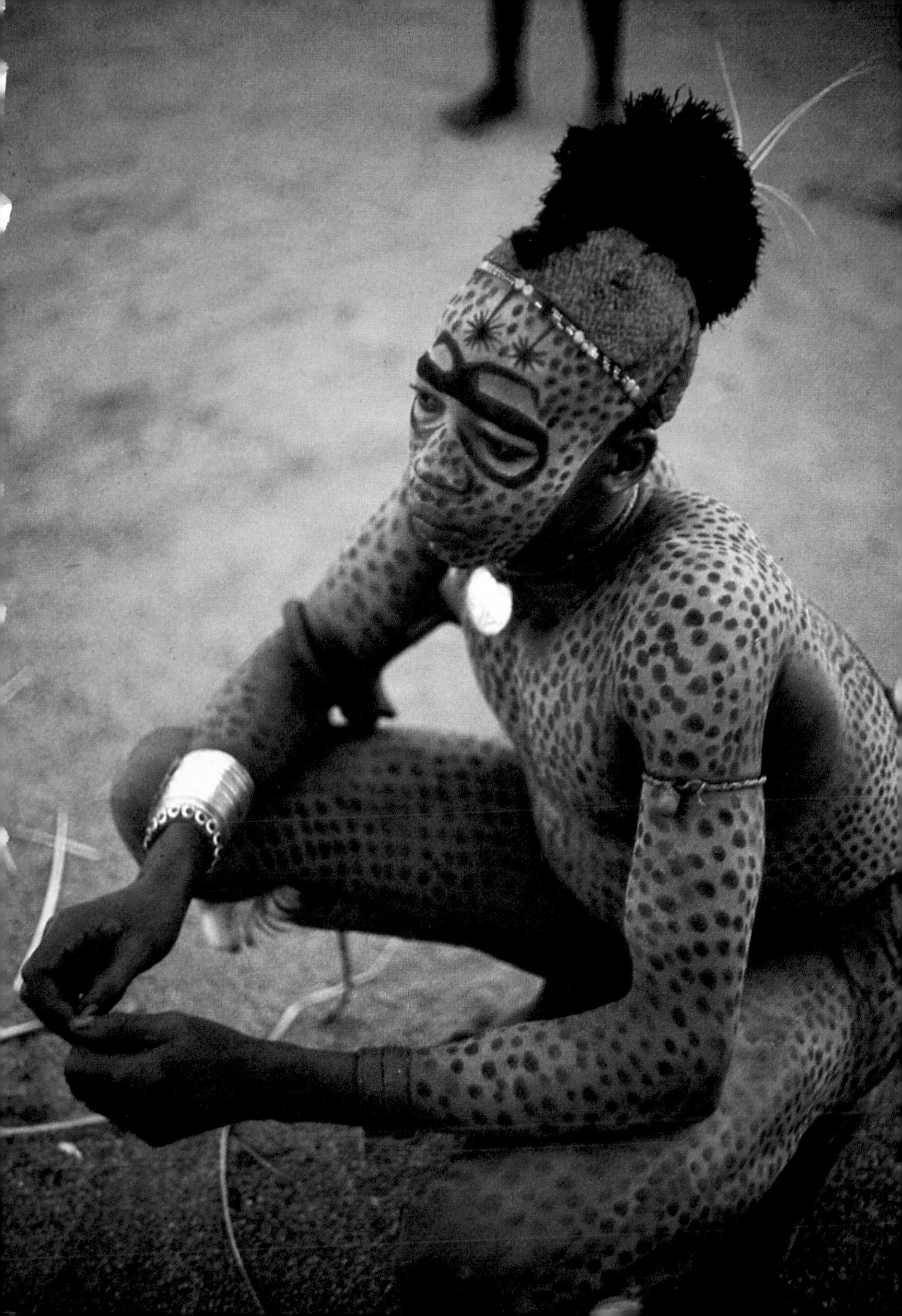

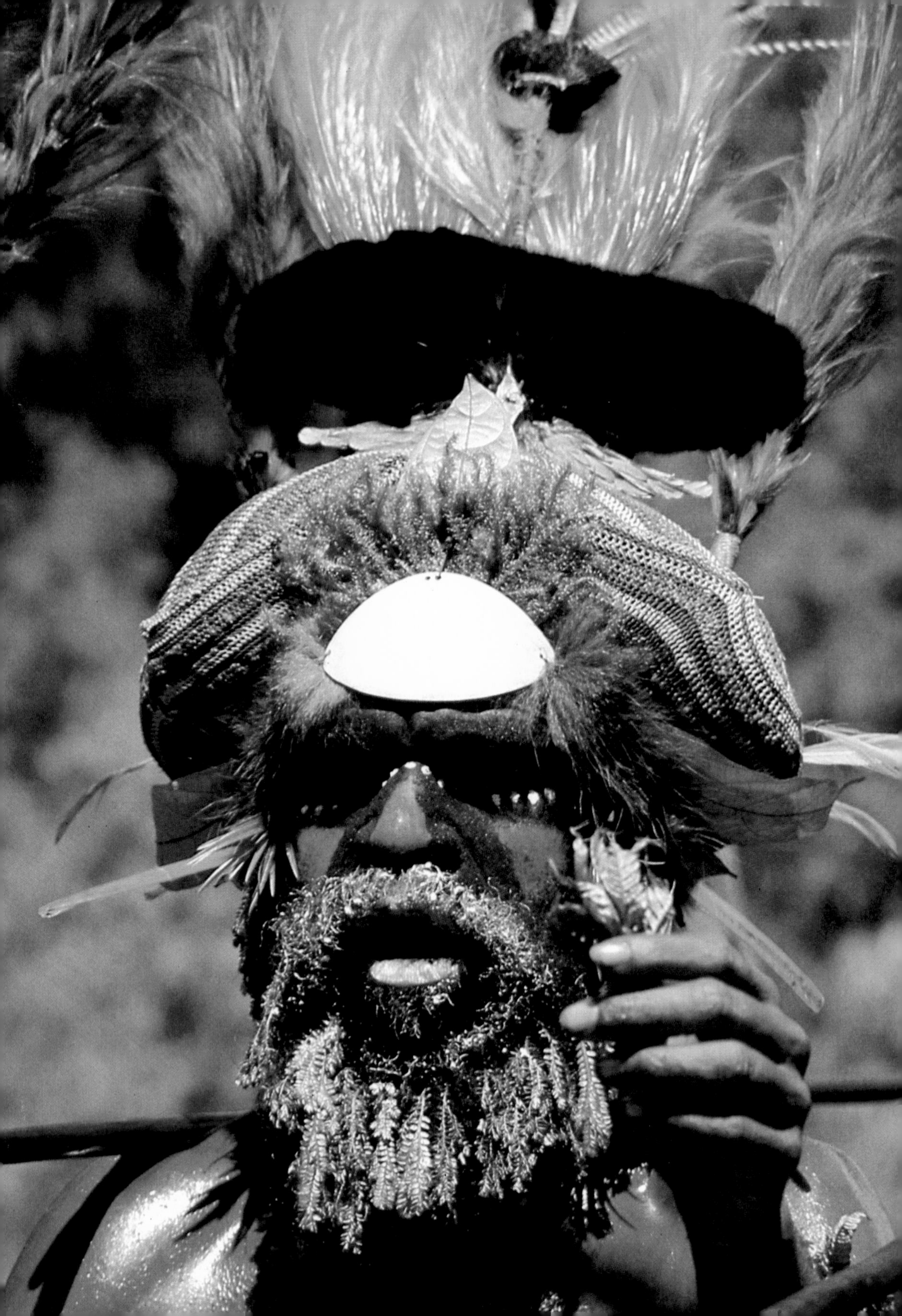

*Each item of the elaborate decoration of this Mount Hagen man (New Guinea) is chosen for its aesthetic or symbolic significance.*

BODY ART, like any other art form, ranges from the frivolous to the serious. Among the Bangwa of Cameroon the body is painted and otherwise decorated for a number of reasons. Sometimes it is purely cosmetic—body art for body art's sake. Both men and women care for their skin and their hair, washing and oiling them and buying their preparations in the market: sticky balls of leaves, powdered barks, and fragrant woods. All are pounded together and mixed, then rubbed into the body and hair to make them shine.

At other times they cover their bodies with the gold-red powder of camwood. In this fashion they celebrate births and marriages, the crowning of their chiefs and the ritual fattening of adolescent girls. Red is the colour of life, of celebration and of joy.

At funerals the bodies of the mourners are painted with dark clays, whose colour and patterning indicate the wearer's relationship to the dead person.

Body decoration among the Bangwa also indicates status. Royals have special scarification (or cicatrization) marks on their chests and backs, which are not allowed to commoners. Likewise, slaves and retainers have special marks or wear certain ornaments. A beautiful woman has her ears pierced, her teeth filed and her stomach scarified, while a handsome man has lustrous black hair (which is dyed if it begins to fade), a strong, shining, preferably stout body, a peaked hairstyle and the ornaments of his class. Twins, mothers and fathers of twins, and priests also have their own distinctive forms of body decoration.

Among the Bangwa (with whom I lived for two years), the dividing line between cosmetics and ritual body decoration is not very clear. Are ear piercing and teeth filing aesthetic or ritual in their purpose?

Since the functions of all institutions are multiple, it often happens that one aspect or another becomes stressed through the prejudice of the observer. A case in point is the Andaman Islanders. Do they paint to make themselves beautiful, as one observer insists, or is it to assure themselves of supernatural protection, as another has it?

The Andamaners ornament their bodies with clays and pigments, and the elaborate designs painted on both men and women would seem to have a primarily aesthetic origin. The painting is done by the women, who decorate each other, their husbands and their male relatives, competing with each

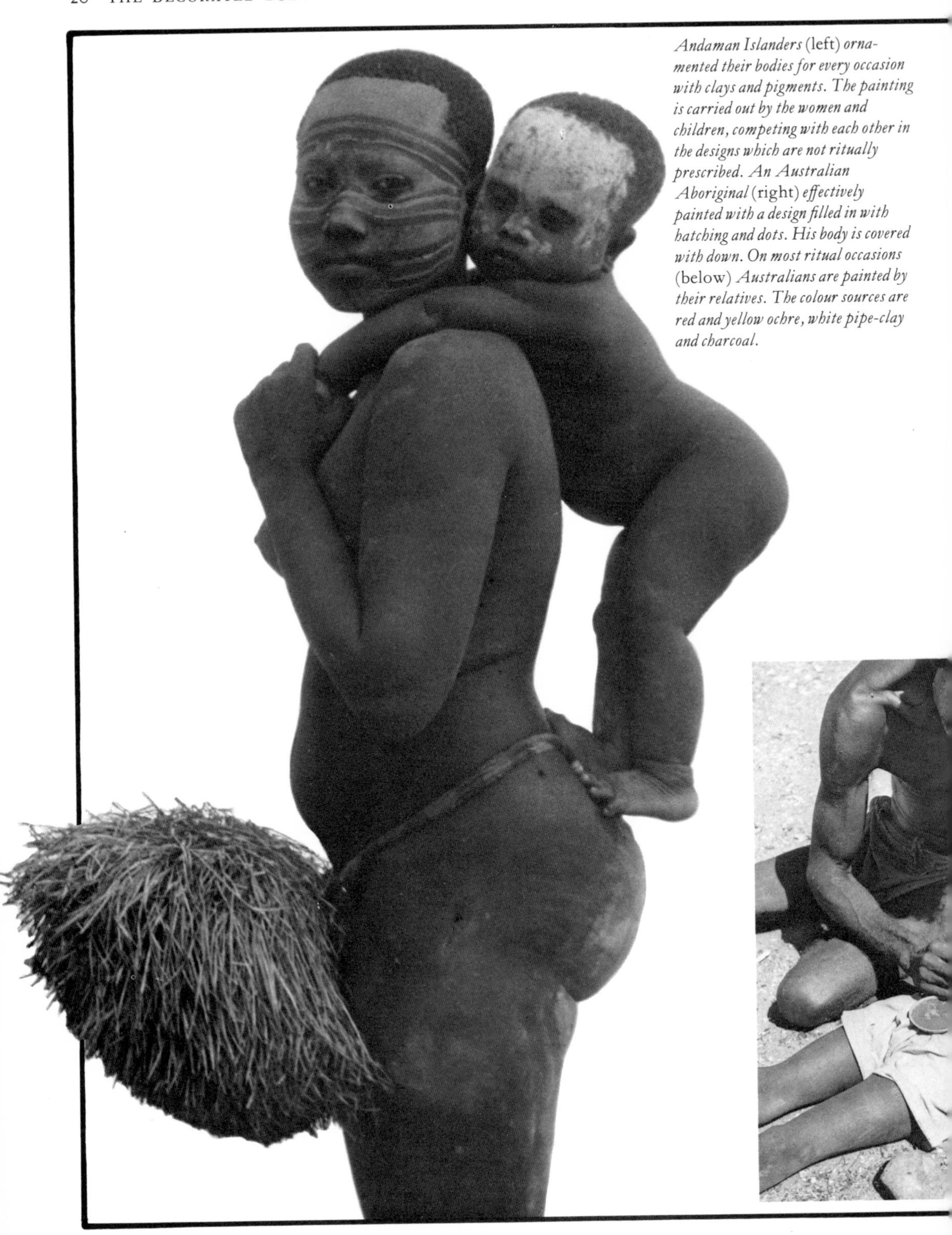

*Andaman Islanders* (left) *ornamented their bodies for every occasion with clays and pigments. The painting is carried out by the women and children, competing with each other in the designs which are not ritually prescribed. An Australian Aboriginal* (right) *effectively painted with a design filled in with hatching and dots. His body is covered with down. On most ritual occasions* (below) *Australians are painted by their relatives. The colour sources are red and yellow ochre, white pipe-clay and charcoal.*

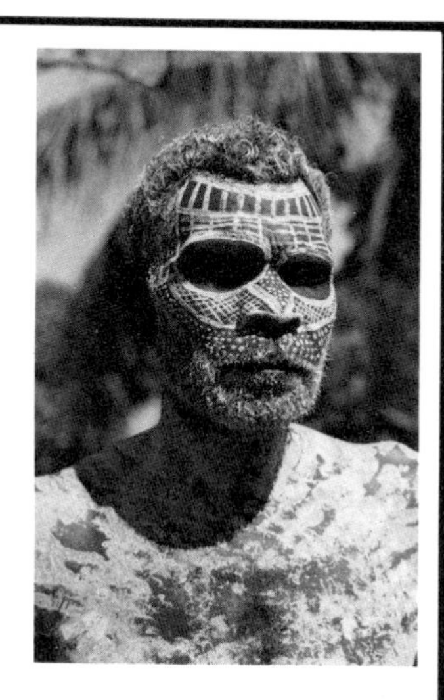

other in the designs, which are not ritually or rigidly prescribed by custom. A successful artistic innovation is copied by others in the same way as fashions in clothes and cosmetics develop and disappear in the West. The women say that they paint their bodies 'to make them look well'.

Yet the Andaman women also paint special patterns for special occasions: feasts, dances and ceremonies. Even a corpse may be painted brightly before it is buried, as in some contemporary Western practices. But for cosmetic or ritual reasons?

The Australians (in this book when I refer to Australians I mean the original inhabitants of the continent, the Black or Aboriginal Australians) paint their bodies as an intensely serious religious function. During rituals, as we shall see, the patterns and colours are set down by tradition and are applied by special persons on special occasions. In everyday behaviour, however, they make themselves attractive by availing themselves of any pattern and any colour. A whole family may spend long leisure hours improving each other's appearance, painting ornate designs on different parts of the body, designs which have no prescribed form and no symbolic meaning: longitudinal parallel bands of red and yellow and black may extend up the legs, back and abdomen, with transverse lines on the chest, shoulders and the outer surface of the thighs, connected here and there by lattice patterns and concentric circles. Parents paint their children, displaying them proudly to other members of the group.

On the Forrest River, in Western Australia, a favourite cosmetic, non-ritual, pattern is a broad step-and-ladder drawn on the front surface of the legs. The design continues up the trunk to the level of the nipples and then circles outwards down an arm on either side to run out at the elbow.

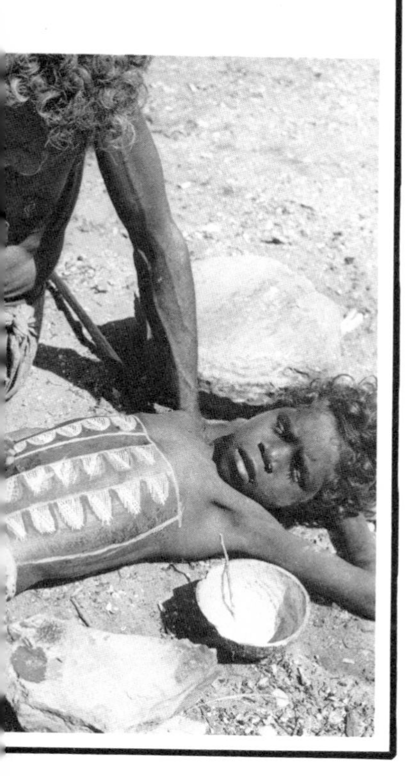

The North American Indians also delighted in transforming the natural body into a work of art appreciated for itself as well as for its ritual and social role. One north-western group, the Haida, painted their faces daily for cosmetic purposes; for dances and ceremonies, ritual designs and colours were more carefully applied and included heraldic crests on foreheads and cheeks. Haida men and women wore ear-pendants and nose-pins and, if high-born, crests were tattooed on their legs and arms. Hair was braided for women but left free and cut across at shoulder length for men. Like the Bangwa, Australians and Andamaners, both sexes spent a lot of time painting and caring for their bodies. The men plucked out their facial and body hair with tweezers and smeared their bodies and head hair with bear-grease and scents.

Unfortunately, the nineteenth century saw the complete disappearance of this specialized and highly developed art of the body in North America, although in some cases a good deal of information has been preserved.

The Thompson Indians were inveterate painters, and we are lucky that the techniques, the designs, their meaning and function were recorded in detail by James A. Teit. Although we must depend on Teit's drawings and on the accounts he heard from old men—much of the complexity of Thompson Indian body painting had disappeared by the time he visited them—his material is plentiful enough for us to get a good picture of their body art.

The Thompson Indians inhabited a plateau between the Rocky Mountains and the Thompson River, where they lived off salmon and also gathered plants and hunted during spring and summer. In the winter, they congregated in one place where they lived off what they had collected. It was in this period of enforced inactivity that they held their ceremonies. Through the long winter, body painting flourished and tattoos were executed.

Most young people painted their faces for cosmetic reasons, experimenting with designs and colours, even changing their face and body patterns several times a day. At puberty, young boys were tattooed, the patterns being made by blackening a thread with powdered charcoal and drawing it under the skin with a needle. Finer needles of bone or cactus spines were used for dots and figures drawn on the skin with wetted charcoal or pricked over with cactus and other thorns. These thorns were tied in small bunches, generally with the points close together.

Tattooing, like painting, had the usual range of functions: ornament, magic, an ordeal to prove courage, initiation rite, preventative against old age and illness, relationship with the guardian spirits, identification, and a property mark on slaves.

But it was at painting that the Thompson Indians excelled. Teit stresses three important features of Thompson Indian culture which had a direct influence on this art. One was the guardian spirit complex, another shamanism, and the third the ghost dance.

The quest for a guardian spirit was open to all Thompson

Indians. It was only obligatory for men, however, women having the choice of obtaining a spirit helper or not. Boys were encouraged to go out before puberty, keeping a series of one-night vigils in order to make contact with a spirit which would appear in a vision or during a dream-like state. The identity of guardian spirits, often represented in body paintings, includes the sun, the moon, the stars, sunsets, thunder, rain, the rainbow, snow, water, the coyote, the otter, the weasel, the raven, the cedar, the fir, and tobacco. They could bring success in gambling, control of the weather during hunting, imperviousness to wounds and to certain illnesses. An individual could have three, four or even more guardian spirits.

During the winter dances, the men sang their guardian spirit songs and the audience appeared painted all over with red. The singers and dancers painted individually, using all kinds of patterns and the whole gamut of colours available. The designs represented the individual's guardian spirit, the spirit having indicated to him the designs to paint.

Each person acquired a guardian spirit during initiation ceremonies, and took on the qualities with which the guardian spirit was endowed. Shamans had exclusive rights to the spirits of the night, the sky, parts of the body and the bat. Hunters and fishermen, women and gamblers, had specially relevant guardian spirits. A man with deer power could run as fast as a deer and take deer easily.

Apart from its own appropriate paintings, each guardian spirit had designs which it advised people to paint in order to cure illness or ward off a mood. Thus one woman, when she was widowed, painted the upper part of her forehead red and the lower part yellow. Below each eye were four vertical lines of medium length. Her hair up to the place where it was cut as a sign of widowhood was painted red. The brow painting represented the day and dawn and the lines below the eyes were tears. Body painting thus had value for individuals as a therapeutic aid in times of personal distress.

The sun and its attributes were the special guardian spirits of warriors, and the Thompson Indians, a relatively peace-loving community, sought their help when they took to the warpath. Before going to war, the men stayed for several days in their sweatbath, praying to their guardians for protection and painting their bodies. While the men were away, the women danced, sang and painted their faces to ensure victory. Each warrior had an individual pattern, though nobody had the *right* to wear black unless he had killed an enemy; but occasionally a person advertised his *intention* of killing by wearing black.

A common warrior's design for the face was half red half black. Another was alternating stripes of red and black covering the chin and jawbone. The black stripes may have indicated the number of people he had killed in his lifetime.

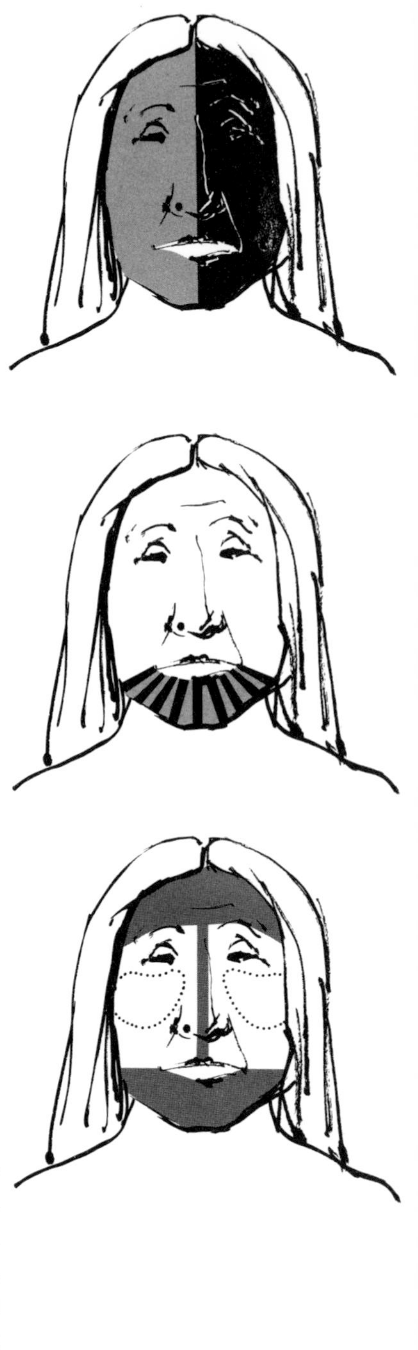

For the war dance ceremonies a famous warrior decorated himself in the following manner. He was naked except for a plain buckskin breechclout, a necklace and a headband fashioned from the skin of a grizzly bear. The claws of the feet projected from it at either side. Two large eagle tail feathers were attached to the headband and daubed red. His back hair was tied up in a knot behind the neck, while in the front it was stiffened with clay into a pointed horn. This was painted red, apart from a black ring around the middle. At each side of the base a white spot was painted. His brow was painted with two narrow horizontal lines and both ears were red, while a narrow red line ran under each eye. On his face a raven was painted in solid black, the beak extending up between the eyes, the body covering the nose and upper lip, and the wings spread out on the cheeks. The tail consisted of five diverging lines on his chin. Symbols of two black snakes were drawn vertically on the left side of the cheek, and a symbol of the sun, also in black, on the right. The right arm below the elbow, including the hand, was red. On his left arm above the elbow were two parallel rings in black, the space between being filled with vertical lines in red and black. His ribs were painted alternately red and black, and a red streak extended down his backbone from the nape of the neck to the small of the back. His left foot and his right foot and leg from the knee down were painted black. His necklace consisted of grizzly bear claws attached to a strip of fur. The grizzly bear, the eagle and the raven were known to be this warrior's guardian spirits. The other designs are to be explained as follows: the painting on the brow represented clouds; the rib design on the chest and back were typical warriors' patterns; an amulet was painted on the left arm. The red below the eyes and ears brought good luck in hearing and seeing. The painting on the right arm meant blood. The black painting of the lower legs and feet was practical, since it helped concealment when approaching the enemy.

In all the paintings, the main idea was to bring luck (red) to the warrior and ill luck (black) to the adversary.

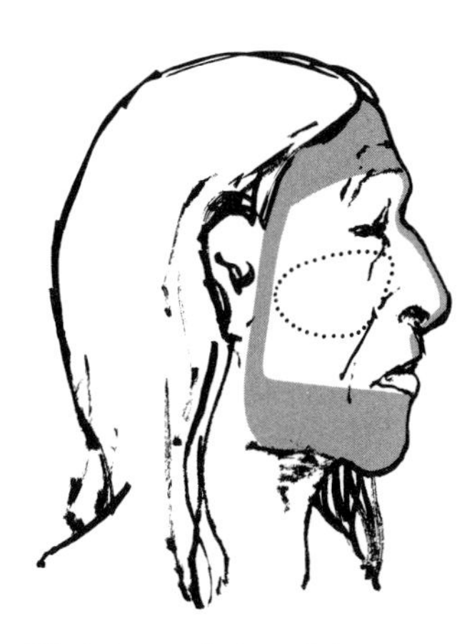

*The designs on the faces of the Thompson Indians represented the individual's guardian spirit. A common warrior's design was half red, half black, the main idea being to bring him luck (red) and his adversary misfortune (black). Another was alternating stripes of black and red covering chin and jawbone, the number of black stripes possibly indicating the number of people he had killed. The guardian spirit might also suggest designs to ward off a mood, as with the widowed woman drawn here (see page 23).*

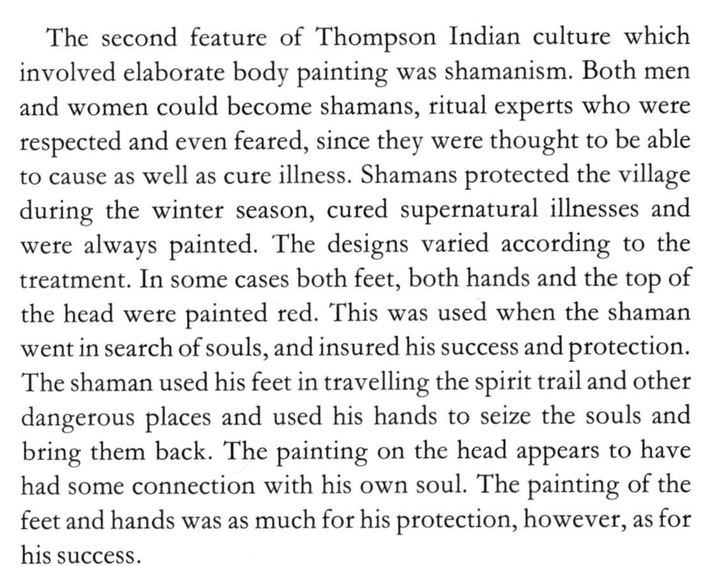

The second feature of Thompson Indian culture which involved elaborate body painting was shamanism. Both men and women could become shamans, ritual experts who were respected and even feared, since they were thought to be able to cause as well as cure illness. Shamans protected the village during the winter season, cured supernatural illnesses and were always painted. The designs varied according to the treatment. In some cases both feet, both hands and the top of the head were painted red. This was used when the shaman went in search of souls, and insured his success and protection. The shaman used his feet in travelling the spirit trail and other dangerous places and used his hands to seize the souls and bring them back. The painting on the head appears to have had some connection with his own soul. The painting of the feet and hands was as much for his protection, however, as for his success.

As part of their cure, shamans prescribed painting for their patients. Most of the designs were derived from the dreams of the shaman and were similar in character to the dream and shaman designs mentioned above. Some were different: spots could be painted over places where there was pain, lines drawn above and below these places, circles around wounds and sores. Sometimes the shaman did the paintings, sometimes the patient or his relatives were told how to do them.

The third feature of the life of Thompson Indians which profoundly influenced their body painting was the public ceremonies and dances, particularly the ghost dances. These dances brightened the long, dark winters, often lasting several days, with a number of separate communities taking part. In the winter they danced in the long winter houses; in the spring they danced outside.

Each dancer had his or her face painted, usually red. Chiefs had perpendicular stripes down the entire length of their cheeks, made by wiping off the colour with the fingertips. Both men and women also used yellow, and alternate stripes of red and white and black.

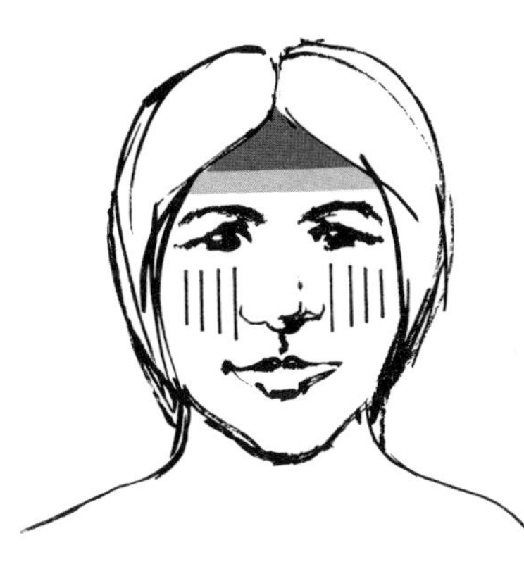

A number of designs were specifically painted for the ghost dances, dances involved with a religion which promised the American Indians a restoration of the old forms of life, the expulsion of the white invaders and the return of the deceased ancestors, the ghosts. Originating with the Paiute Indians at Walker Lake, Nevada, this religion reached the Thompson Indians in the last quarter of the nineteenth century. A number of patterns were specifically designed for the dances, usually involving stripes and designs symbolic of celestial bodies. Many of the designs had reference to prayers, speech, sight and hearing. Circles around the eyes, for example, indicated seeing, and the person used this design to increase his visionary powers.

A noted chief of the ghost dances painted in the following way. A red stripe extended across the upper part of the forehead and the whole chin was painted red. The chin design represented cumulus clouds, the brow design cirrus. On his naked body he had a triangular figure composed of two red lines commencing one on each side of the neck and uniting at the stomach. Between these there were six or eight horizontal lines equal distances apart. The upper left arm and the right forearm, including the wrist, the thumb and the back of the hand and fingers, were painted red, representing the shadows of mountains and one of his guardian spirits. He had a red ring around each leg, below the knee, and numerous red stripes extending from it to the ankles, all around the legs. This design was supposed to represent the fringes of leggings.

Even though we have no contemporary photographs and most of the material is based on informants' memories, it is clear that the Thompson Indians, along with hundreds of other Indian groups, had an elaborate system of painting, involving their social life, their cosmology and their symbolism.

Body painting was an art in which the ornamental designs were complex and effective and had a deep meaning. The colours used by the Thompson Indians were red, yellow, blue, white and black. (I shall discuss colour symbolism in the 'Symbolic Body' chapter.) They also used a powdered micaceous hematite which gave the body a shiny, sparkling appearance. The paint was sometimes applied dry, but usually, particularly for the very fine work, the designs were applied with the colours mixed with water or grease. Some designs were made by painting the skin with one colour and then scraping the paint off with teeth or pieces of shell. As a rule, individuals painted themselves, though there were experts. Water or sheets of mica were used as looking glasses.

Painting was a serious matter and everyone took an interest in the correct application of patterns. Most people carried small bags of paint attached to their belts, and replenished them from larger ones kept at home. Rough skin was well rubbed and painted with pencils of deer's back fat. Dry red paint was rubbed on the face and hands in cold weather to keep out the cold and prevent freezing. Black circles were made around the eyes to shade them and prevent injuries from the glare of a strong sun or bright snow. Painting therefore served practical as well as symbolic, religious ends.

The major interest of Thompson Indian designs, however, is the complex meanings attached to colours and shapes. Some designs were used by men, by hunters or warriors; others were used by both sexes. Some designs had religious significance, but none had an exclusive meaning, so that a blue spot indicating an ancestor could be a decorative mark in another context.

Teit wrote:

> Much of it was for ornament, but much also had a strong connection with religion, dreams, guardian spirits, cure of disease, protection, prayers, speech, good luck, war or death. It was often difficult to distinguish between a painting used purely for ornament and one having other significance. Almost the same symbols or designs and colours were used in all cases. As a rule middle-aged and old people painted less for ornament than young people. If young people painted with small elaborate designs in various colours it was usually for ornament and to fascinate the opposite sex. . . . Among elderly people, as a rule, representations of dreams alone were painted and nothing added for mere ornament.

While body painting has virtually disappeared as a living art among the North American Indians, in South America it still flourishes among the more remote tribes, but on the whole contact with Europeans has rung its death knell. Just as anthropologists were beginning to understand that painting conferred upon people part of their essential dignity as human beings, and art historians were beginning to consider body painting as art, it was too late. The painted ones looked with disdain at the pale-faced, naked Europeans, but unable to explain the importance and aesthetic value of their art, slowly or quickly abandoned it.

In South America, in the nineteenth century, Europeans expressed amazement, shock, scientific interest or intolerance when confronted with the splendidly painted Indians. I have already noted Darwin's comments on the Fuegians. Dobrizhoffer described the Abipoines of Paraguay as savages 'who increased their frightful appearance which nature had given them by certain adscititious ornaments, one of these being to stain their hair with purple juice or the blood of oxen'. Alfred Wallace, who like Darwin visited South America in the middle of the century, made journeys up the Rio Negro and the Amazon and commented on the men and women who danced for his party. They were adorned in diamond patterns, their entire bodies painted in brilliant hues, purple, blue and black predominating, with red and yellow pointings to the designs and their faces striped or spotted red, the ears thickly lacquered, and stripes drawn down their necks and shoulders 'like ochre collars and epaulettes'.

As far as the missionaries were concerned, body painting was magic, pagan and to be stamped out. Moreover, unconsciously imbued with a busy, capitalistic ethic, they were dismayed by the long hours the Indians spent cosseting, oiling and painting the dangerous and sinful human body, when they should be fishing, farming or hunting. Body painting was magic and as magic it could not be art. Yet the fact that the body was painted for the enjoyment of the individual and his friends must have been obvious to a casual observer. In 1857, for example, when the warship *Maracanha* made its first appearance on the Paraguay River, a party of Indians paid her a visit; and on the following day they were seen to have drawn anchors all over their bodies. One man covered the upper half of his body with a representation of a European officer, complete with buttons, stripes, belt and coat-tails. This must surely have been art for art's sake.

After the bigoted, slightly nervous reactions of missionaries and administrators it is a pleasure to read a more sympathetic account of one South American society, the Caduveo, and look at their body art from a comprehensive, anthropological point of view.

The Caduveo, along with the Toba and Pilaga of Paraguay, are the few remnants of the great Mbaya-Guaicuru peoples. In the seventeenth century, the Mbaya-Guaicuru, superbly dressed and ornamented, had their kings and queens, nobles who delighted in tournaments and war and were freed from all menial tasks by a slave group, the Guana, who tilled the soil and paid their lords a tribute of farm produce in exchange for protection. The Mbaya nobles wore the mark of their rank on their bodies, pictorial designs either painted or tattooed. They also plucked out their facial hair, including eyebrows and eyelashes, and compared their hairy European con-

*North American Indians once wore elaborate body decoration. The nineteenth century saw the complete disappearance of this specialized and highly developed art, and today, as for the Hopi Indian* (right) *from Arizona, the meanings are largely forgotten. The fine painting on the legs and arms of the Tukano boy* (below) *from the north-west Amazon can be seen being applied by a wife to her husband's legs* (below right). *For the Tukano, an unpainted man is a naked man.*

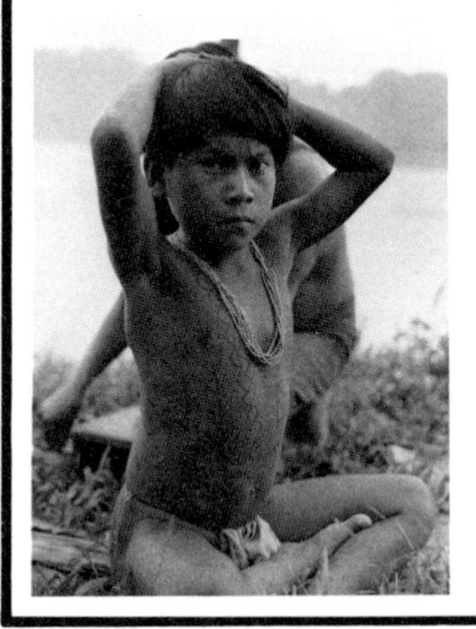

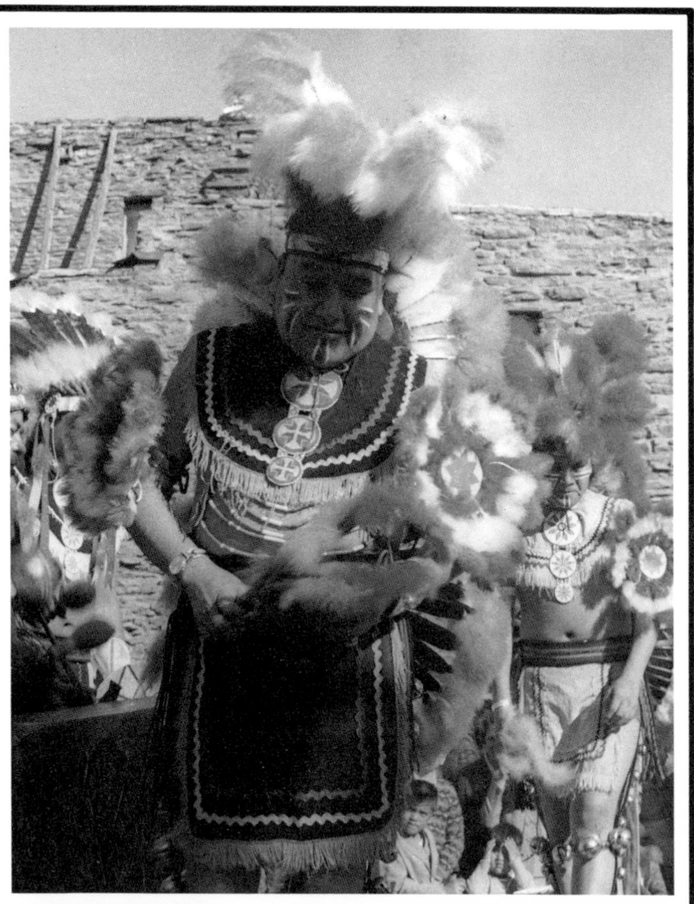

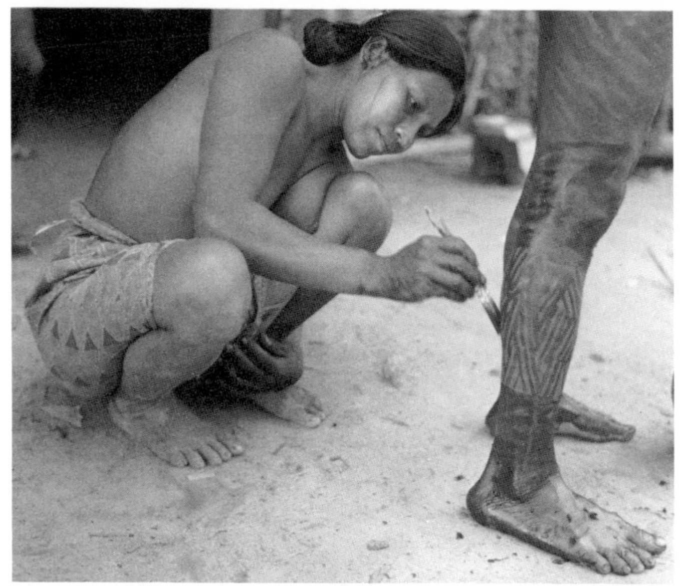

querors to rheas. Too proud to procreate—abortion and infanticide were almost routine—they ensured the continuance of their race and class by adopting young prisoners-of-war, who were fostered by lower-class families and occasionally visited their own families. Until the age of fourteen they were painted black and called by the name Indians used for Negroes.

In the Mbaya community body painting was carried out by women. The face, and sometimes the whole body, was covered with an interlacing of arabesques alternating with geometric motifs. Nobles had only their foreheads painted; an entirely painted face was the mark of a commoner. Today the Caduveo still paint their bodies, for their own pleasure and for erotic purposes, the paintings reinforcing the contours of the body and creating a provocative effect. The technique has apparently remained unchanged over the centuries. The artist, still a woman, uses a fine bamboo spatula dipped in the juice of a plant which begins by being colourless and through oxidation becomes blue-black. She places the design on her living model with neither sketch nor prototype to guide her. The paintings are renewed every few days.

Caduveo body designs are complex, improvised on a set of traditional or classical themes. They are always different, since there is an infinite variety in the arrangement of the basic elements—the spirals, the hatching, the volutes, tendrils and crosses.

> The design is built symmetrically in relation to two linear axes, one of them vertical, following the median plane of the face, the other horizontal, dividing the face at eye level. The eyes are schematically represented on a reduced scale. They are used as starting points for two inverted spirals, one of which covers the right cheek and the other the left side of the forehead.

The Caduveo artist ornaments the upper lips with a bow-shaped motif finished off with a spiral at either end. She makes a design which divides the face in two like the *moko* artist, but here the division is both vertical and horizontal so that the face is marked off into quarters. She applies arabesques to these halves or quarters, irrespective of the position of the nose, the eyes, the cheeks, the forehead and the chin—just as if she were working on a flat unbroken surface.

*Some examples of the complex Caduveo facial paint patterns, showing how the vertical and horizontal axes intersect and divide the face into four symmetrical sections based on an apparent asymmetry.*

The interesting fact about the face paintings of the Caduveo is that there is a symmetry based on an apparent asymmetry: the two axes intersect and divide the face into four sections, the opposite triangles having a symmetrical design. Sometimes the artist accomplishes an image of the face *on the face* by a method of split representation, dividing the face into two profiles and four quarters. This, as Claude Levi-Strauss points out, is a technique used on the north-west coast of America by Indian artists. North-west coast paintings of animals often look as if the animal's face is conceived as a body painting, removed from the body and opened out in a remarkable example of split representation. The animals are represented on flat surfaces and look very similar to the paintings of the Caduveo women. This distinctive technique of splitting the image and pulling the two halves apart is also very similar to the Maori *moko* tattoos, described later, when they are drawn on paper by their 'owners'; and it is found in Ancient Chinese art.

Caduveo face painting and *moko* design in a sense dislocate the face in the interests of their art. The integrity of the face is respected in so far as it cannot be taken apart or flattened, but the natural harmony of the features is of less importance than the artificial harmony of the design. The Caduveo painter,

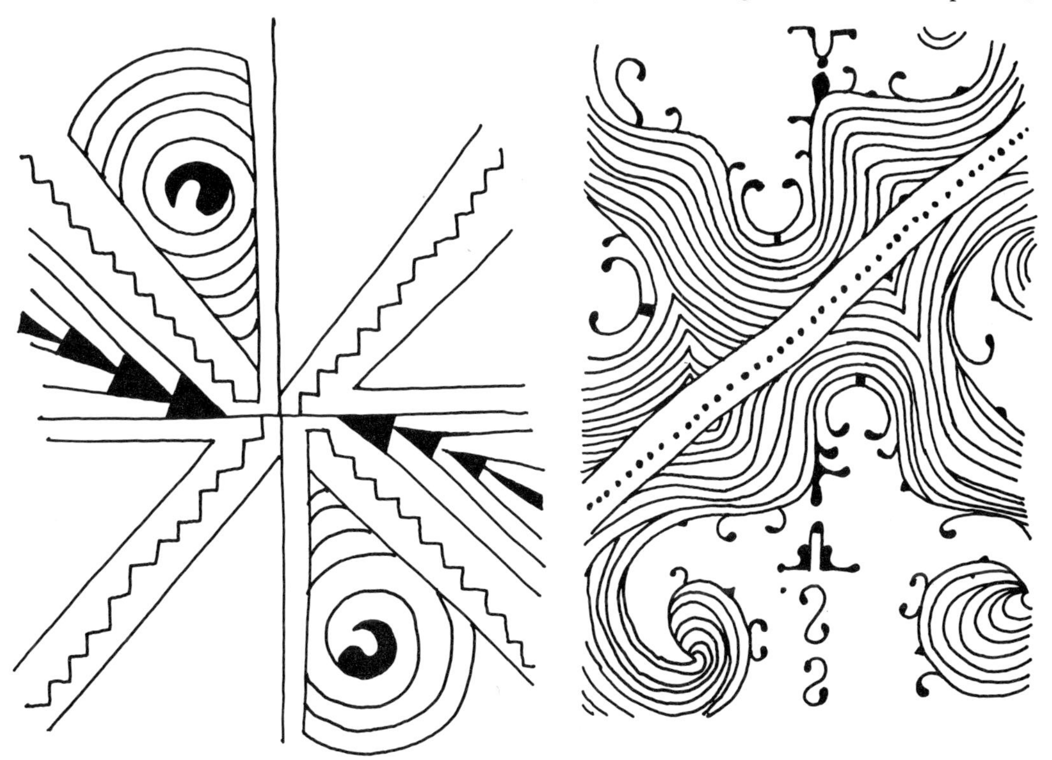

asked to draw the design on a flat surface, draws not the face but the design, respecting its true proportions as if they were painted on a curved surface. To respect the face, she would have to distort the design, as in a Western photograph.

In New Guinea this century, two British anthropologists, Andrew and Marilyn Strathern, have studied another complex form of body decoration, that of the Hageners in the highlands. Men and women paint and decorate their bodies in an equally elaborate and meaningful way, sometimes lightheartedly during courting parties and social visits, but often with a deeper religious meaning which indicates individual and group relationships to ancestors and other spirits. While in other parts of New Guinea art objects are carved and painted as representations of ancestors and reflections of community values, the Hageners, like the Thompson Indians, communicate mostly through body decoration, which as a result is forced to carry a much higher symbolic content and aesthetic interest.

The Hageners and the Hagen area take their name from a 13,000ft mountain in the Western Highlands of New Guinea. They were 'discovered' by the West in the 1930s, when gold prospectors, administrators and missionaries, mainly from Australia, first made their way over the high ranges. Today, the Hageners who live around the administrative centre, Mount Hagen town, number about ninety thousand.

Hagen decoration reflects the competitive nature of their society. They have no hereditary chiefs, and self-made leaders continually compete for temporary advantage over each other. This competition takes place in elaborate ceremonial exchanges, when groups try to outdo each other by the size of their gifts of shell valuables and pigs. Body decoration is applied and decoration worn for temporary displays during which the success of a certain group or an ambitious individual is boastfully paraded. On these political and ceremonial occasions the preparation of the body is of great importance and may take as much time as that actually spent putting on the dances and the cult performances.

The purpose of Hagen decoration is to impress the spectators and rival groups. Weeks of practice precede the final display, and on each new day of dancing a fresh collection of ornaments is assembled. Men begin decorating at dawn, donning their large wigs, aprons and a rear covering of leaves. Feathers are arranged, sprigs of leaves and ferns adjusted, and

*Around Mount Hagen, New Guinea, ochre provides the popular red colour. The wet ochre clay is extracted, wrapped in leaves* (top) *and baked over a fire* (centre). *The baked ochre is then removed from the ashes and placed on a leaf receptacle. Finally the quality of the colour, which is all important, is tried out* (bottom).

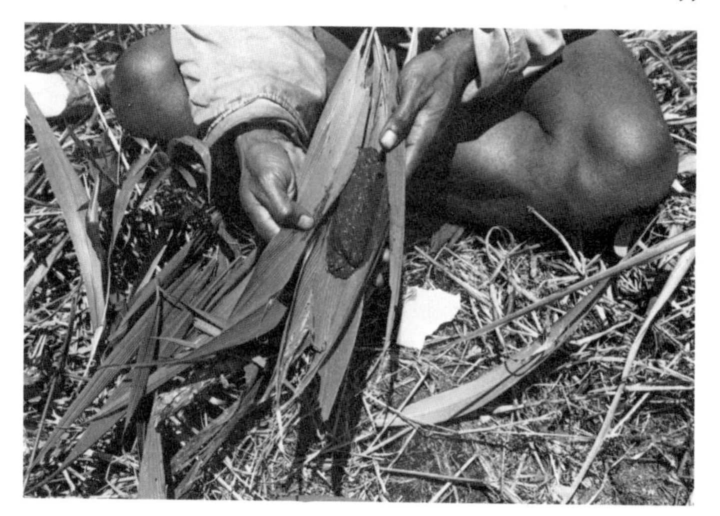

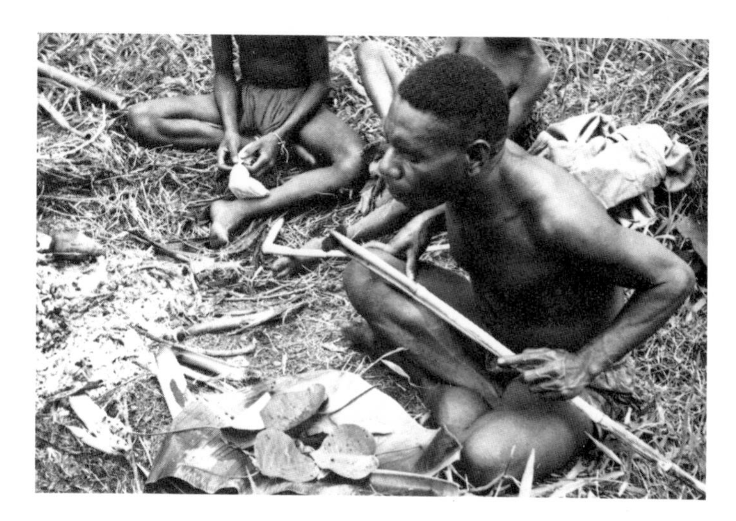

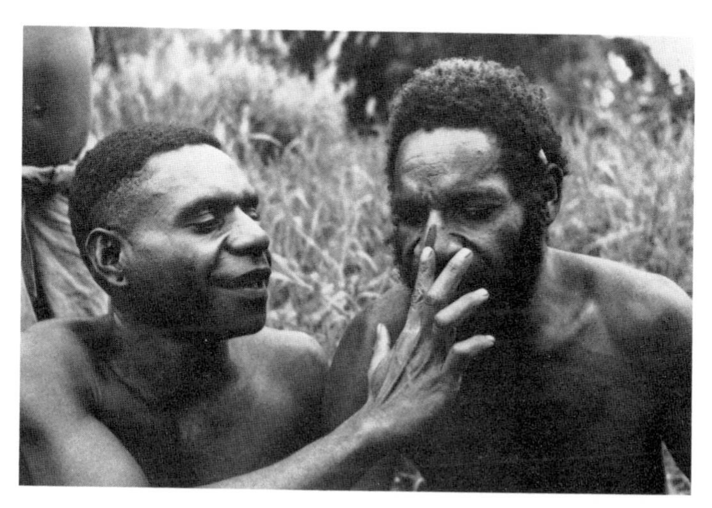

the dancing apron smoothed into place. The most tedious task is the face painting, which requires the help of friends and wives, although mirrors make the job easier today. Assistants mix charcoal with fat or water, smoothing it on the body. Areas where the coloured paint is to be applied are left free, although white paint is sometimes applied directly over the charcoal. Paint brushes are fashioned from twigs with soft leaf swabs at one end which are dipped in the colours.

*Among the Australian Aborigines mourning paint is worn on the body by husband and child, the colours being set by tradition and applied by special persons on special occasions.*

During the dances presents are exchanged and the 'big men' entertain their relatives and visitors with gifts of pork. The dancers are specially looked after and at the same time they are carefully scrutinized by the audience. They comment on the traditional patterns and the individual experiments and innovations. Groups are praised who have the most satisfactory combination of shell decoration, plumes and furs, wigs and aprons and other accessories, but these fall outside the scope of this book and I shall concentrate mainly on the practice and meaning of body painting among the Hageners.

In Hagen society both men and women rub their skin to make it shine. Liquid pig fat is scooped into bamboo tubes and gourd flasks after the cooked pork is removed from the earth ovens; and oil is squeezed from the red and yellow pandanus fruits. Earth paints are white, blue or yellow clays, which are common beside rivers. They are used as powdered pigments. Red ochre powder is scarcer and found only at a few sites, the raw material being a rusty brown clay. This clay is wrapped in leaves and baked on a wooden trestle over a fire, the men turning the packs with special tongs. When the fire dies down, the clay is broken open and the reddest portions are used for the pigment.

The Hageners decorate themselves for everyday business, courting parties, dances and the exchange ceremonies and religious cults. Only at funerals is painting out of place, although even then the body and face are smeared with mud or clay and sometimes ashes, which are said to make the skin 'bad' and 'dry', creating an opposite effect to the shining and beautiful paints and greases. Even at work-parties, when two groups may vie with each other to heave a tree trunk or dig a section of road, body painting is *de rigueur*. Individual men paint their faces, adding outlines in colour around the eyes, the nose and the mouth so that no two men are alike. At elections, meetings and markets, the Hageners dress up; these are informal occasions, when the face is painted in recognition of a public event or to increase sexual attraction.

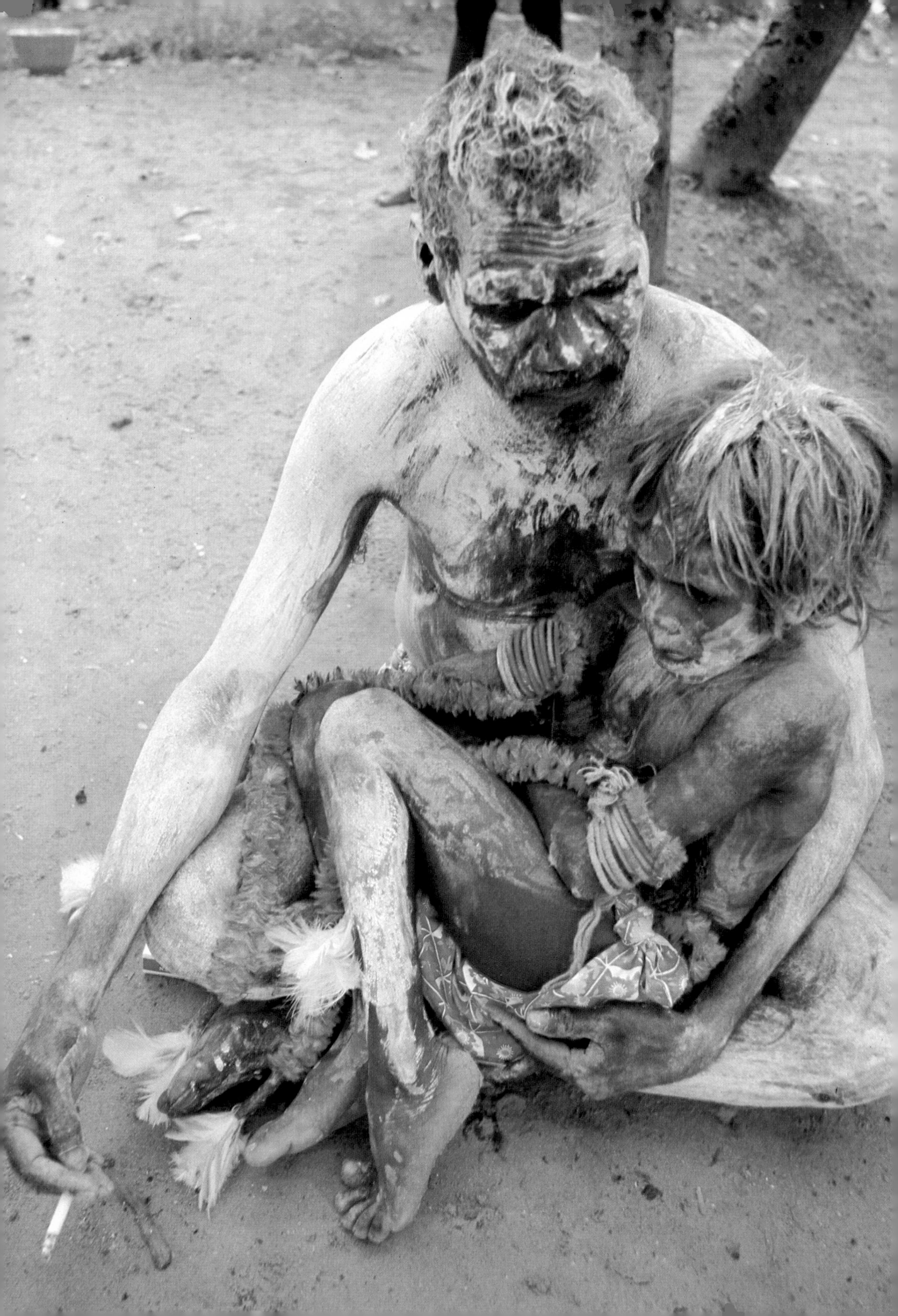

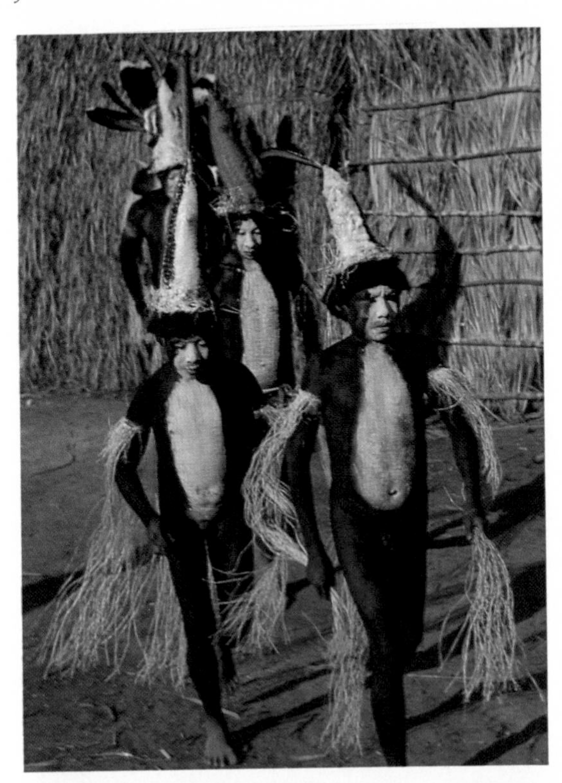

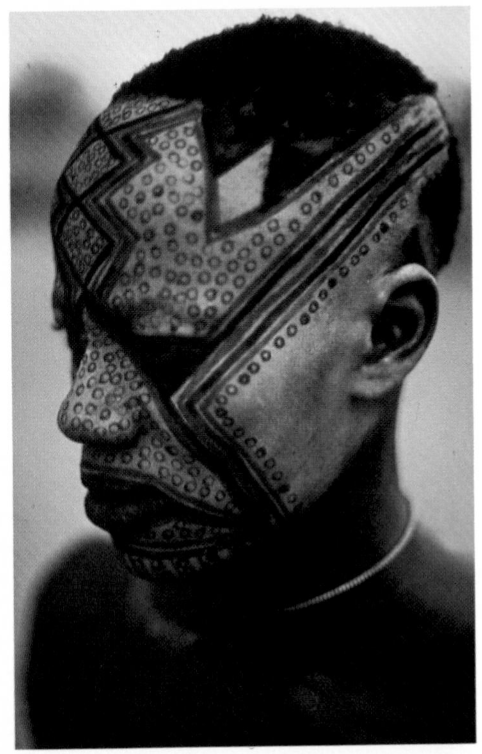

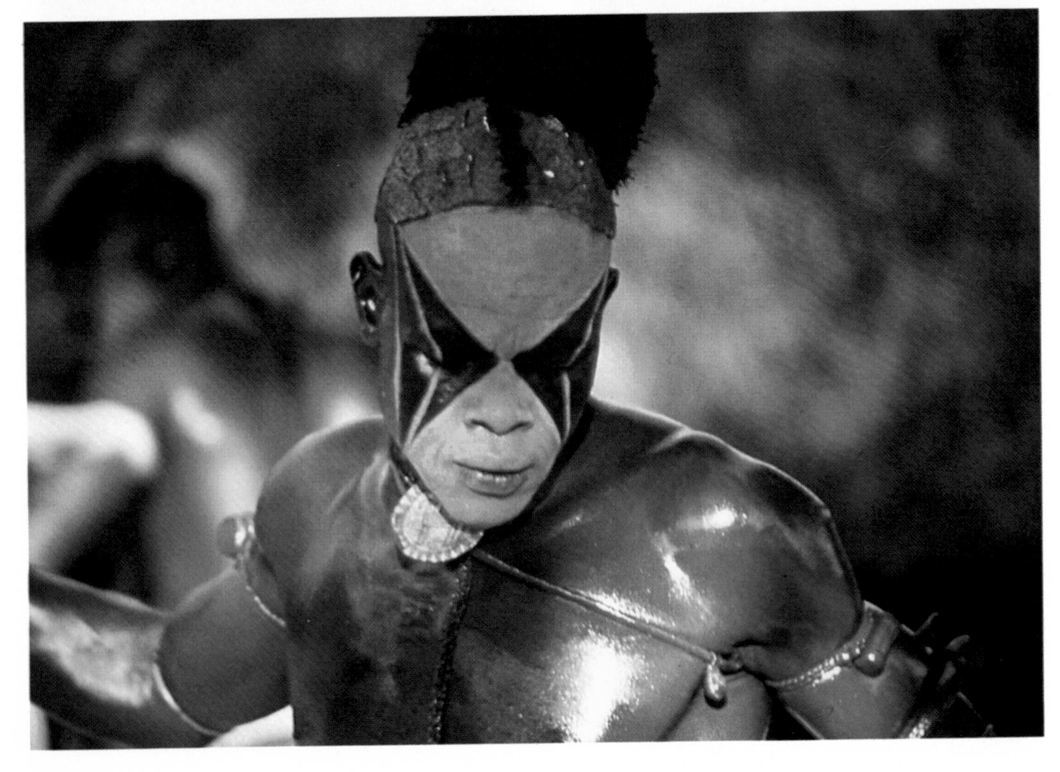

left *Face painting among the Nuba need have no symbolic meaning. It is art for art's sake, the strength of the pattern deriving from symmetrical balance and the juxtaposition of designs and facial features.* far left *Body painting on Txi Kao Indians of Brazil.* below *The facial design of this Nuba youth was inspired by a bird, and bird plumes are attached to his hair. He is decorated for dancing.*

overleaf *A New Guinea Highlander from Mount Hagen prepares himself for a dance, with the aid of a broken mirror and watched by his wife.*

Girls dress up for courting parties, which are held at night in the women's houses. Unmarried girls and young men take part, one or two older women acting as chaperones and watching the dancing. When the men arrive at the courting house they are greeted by the chaperone. The girls stay at the back of the house while the men sing love songs to attract them. Finally the girls emerge and kneel at one end of the room while two men sit cross-legged on either side of them.

> After waving their heads in a stylized preliminary motion, partners press noses together, duck heads down while turning on to the cheek, swing back, turn their heads together twice, retaining contact on the nose and forehead, then duck again. . . . A girl 'turns' alternately with partners on either side of her. . . . Courting is supposed to continue till daylight, when the girls have a right to chase their partners out, threatening them with mud and stinging nettles.

For courting parties the girls are elaborately decorated, wearing, perhaps, a pearl-shell crescent and cowrie necklaces. They are said to mix love-magic with their pigments and the men mix it with their grease, the magic attracting the opposite sex by its perfume. On these occasions the painting of men and women is noticeably different. Women paint their faces in triangles, stipples and streaks of blue, yellow and red, ringing their eyes with white. The men normally use a black base; the designs which follow their facial features are commonly in white, while other colours are found on the cheeks, the chin and the forehead. The white areas are mostly superimposed on the black base, emphasizing the blackness around them. The coloured designs are applied to charcoal-free areas. Blackness, or a combination of black and white, is peculiar to the men; by contrast, the women wear a red base. Boys whose beards have not grown take women's patterns—in fact the charcoal base of the grown men is designed to emphasize the beard and the dark appearance which goes with it.

In both the men's and women's cases the designs on the face are named and individual choice may govern the use of designs on particular occasions, although as we have seen there are limits to personal variation. Two or three young men from a single clan may decide to paint their faces in the same way, but patterns are not rigidly laid down nor are they the property of individual groups or of individuals.

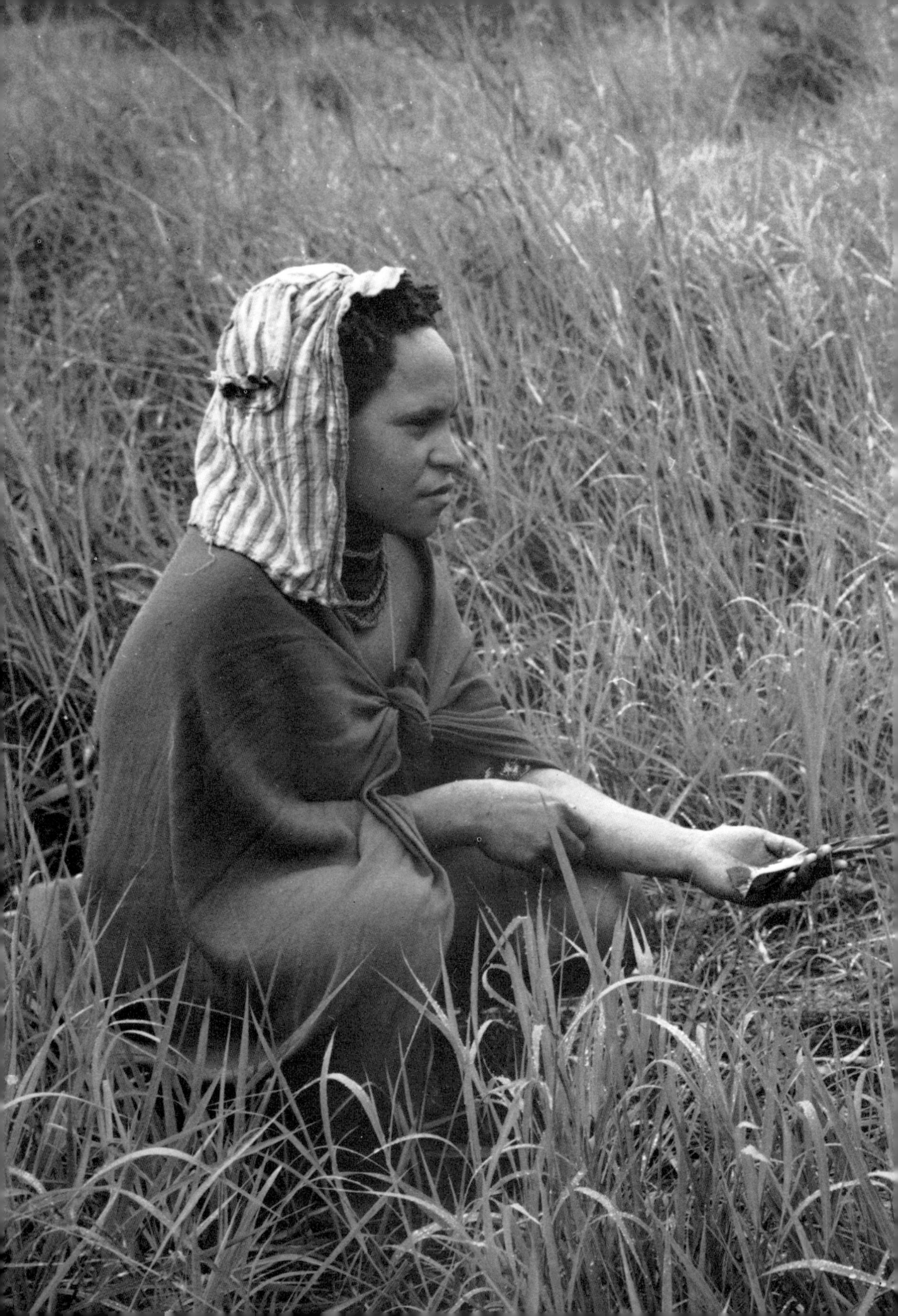

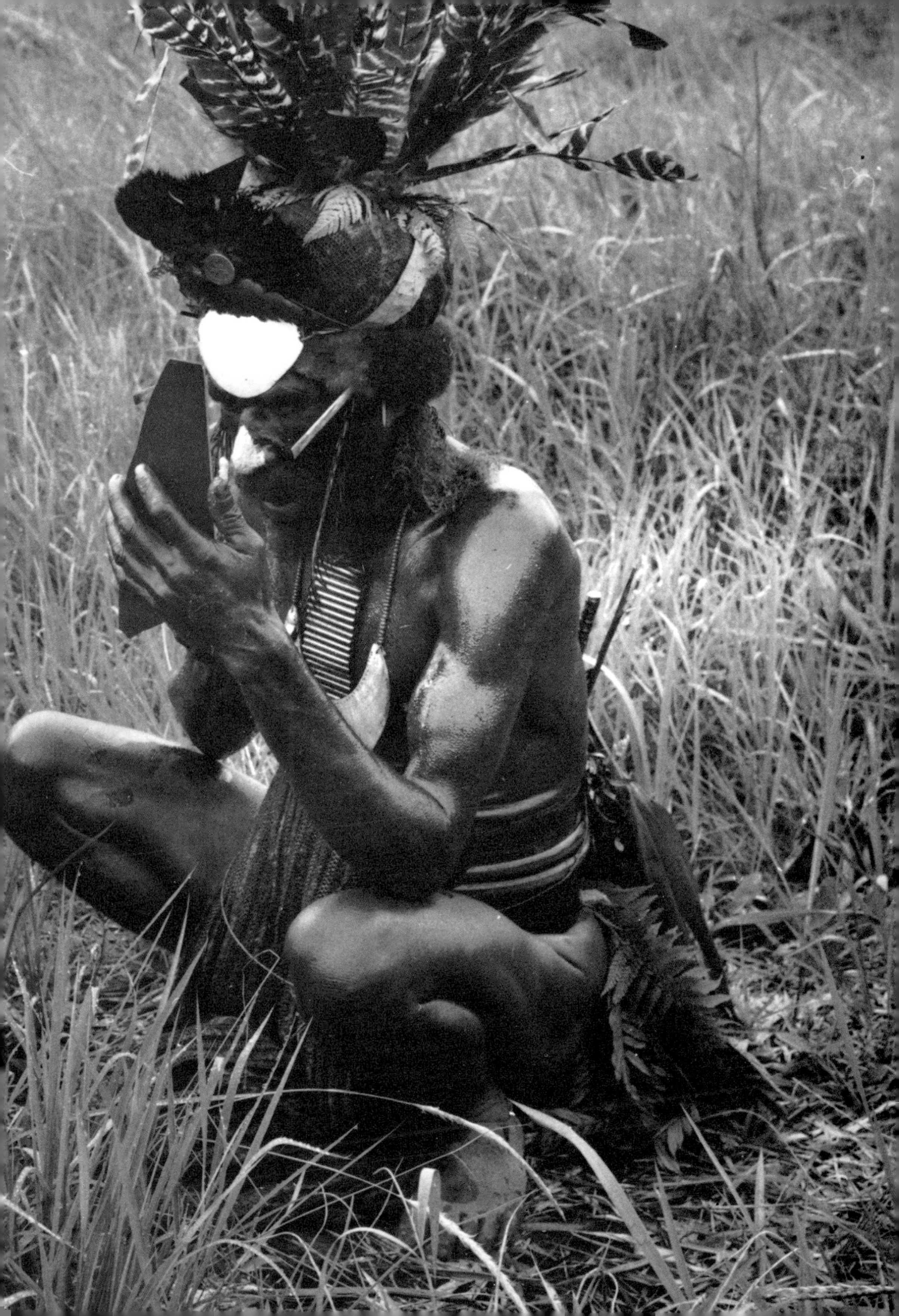

Among all the other reasons for Hagen painting it is inextricably associated with making oneself sexually attractive, and at a deeper level sexual attraction is also linked with a Hagen obsession, the attraction of wealth. For this reason the dancers at an exchange ceremony have to be impressive and attractive. At the ceremonies there is an overall contrast between the white, feature-stressing men's designs on a black background and the brightly coloured ones worn by the women and boys. (This is in sharp contrast to the Thompson Indians where the colours were used equally by men and women.) The men prefer restrained designs with only a limited area of blue, red or yellow. Moreover, the beard is a constraining factor: a man who paints his cheeks applies a single pattern so as not to overshadow his beard. If he encircles his eyes, he does not extend the line in dots and streaks like a woman. The bright elements of a woman's decoration is associated with fertility and friendship, the black and white of the men with aggression.

The Hagen men also wear an impressive type of wig as an element of masculine embellishment. They believe that the ghosts actively lodge in the hair, and a good growth must be evidence of their favour and support. Baldness is a sign that the ghosts have abandoned a man. Wigs are worn as part of the body decoration. In England they are known as 'judges wigs' and they are a kind of canopy of hair and clay which completely surrounds the head and may rest on the shoulders. They are fringed with scarab beetles and marsupial furs and brightly painted with a variety of patterns. The wigs are made by experts who must undergo secret preparations and refrain from sexual intercourse. Hair-cuttings are collected by the owner, usually from other men, while female relatives provide the long ringlets for the side pieces. At the beginning of the 'construction' of a wig a pig is sacrificed to the ancestors and then the work can begin. The whole creation is built up on a frame of pliant cane strips bound with lianas, to which are fastened lengths of hair sewn on with a flying-fox bone. Lumps of wax are allowed to drip on to the wig to set the hair hard. The surface is then smoothed with a round wooden pin and grease rubbed into it before it is painted with bright colours. The fringe of scarab beetles, enclosed in bands of yellow orchid vine, light-coloured ferns and leaves, is added on the day of the dance. These wigs come into their own in a shuffling, twirling dance connected with pig-killing ceremonies, but mainly they are said to attract the women.

*In New Guinea, wigs as well as body painting are worn as an element of masculine embellishment. The wig borne by this young Pialla tribesman is made from human hair and mounted on a bamboo frame.*

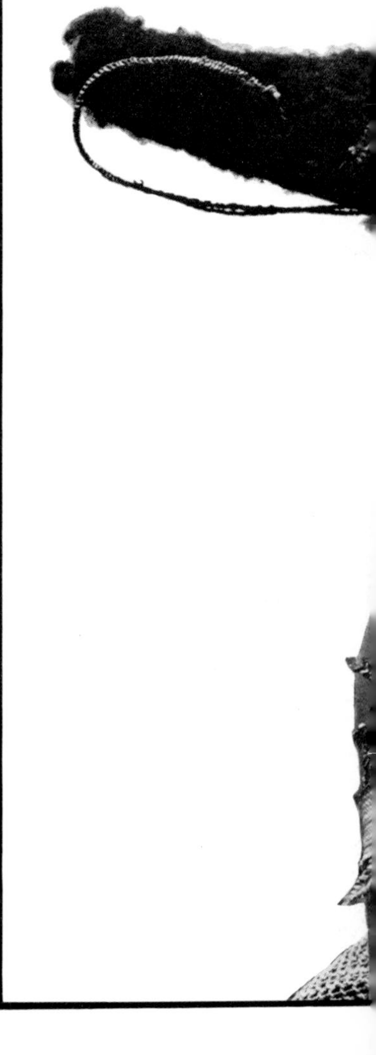

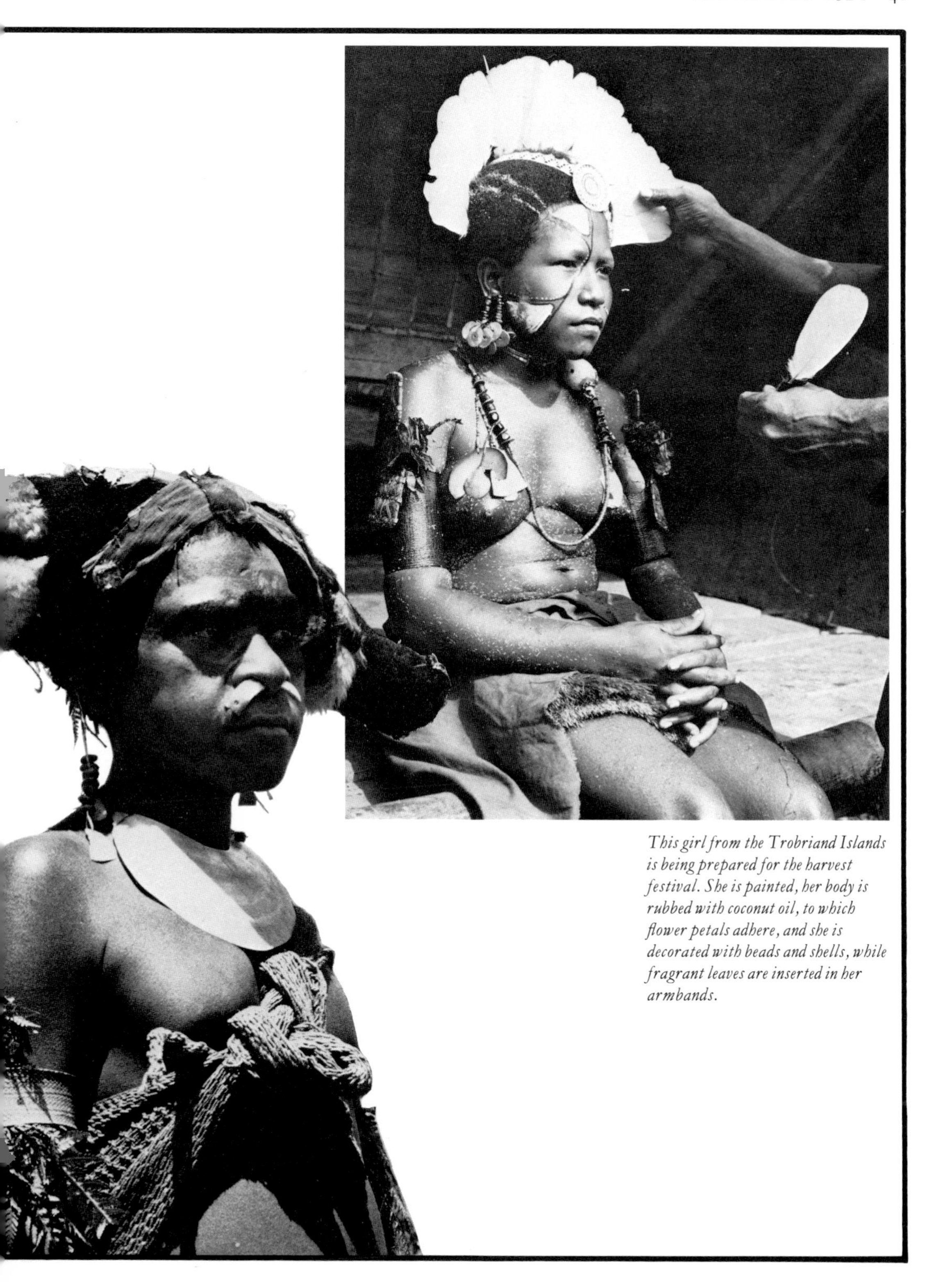

*This girl from the Trobriand Islands is being prepared for the harvest festival. She is painted, her body is rubbed with coconut oil, to which flower petals adhere, and she is decorated with beads and shells, while fragrant leaves are inserted in her armbands.*

In Africa we also find a tradition of personal art motivated by aesthetic and decorative factors based on the human body. With the Thompson Indians the patterns and colours were intimately involved with cultural institutions. In New Guinea, the dark male and bright female elements were linked to a basic opposition between men and women. In both cases the colours and overall decoration made statements about social values.

Among the Sudanese Nuba, the *basis* of their body art rests on a straightforward celebration of the body. Unlike the North American and New Guinean decorations, the brilliant patterns painted on these young men are primarily chosen to complement their physique. Vanity and the wish to attract the attention of other people, particularly of the other sex, are, of course, important elements, but among the Nuba no design may be allowed to hide or detract from the physical form itself, since they stress values associated with the young male body, and demand and reward physical strength, prowess and beauty.

The Nuba (particularly the south-eastern Nuba described by the anthropologist Faris) live in the Kordofan Province of the Democratic Republic of Sudan, where there is a long history of body painting. This brilliant art has survived in an area where government and missionary prejudices against body decoration were not enforced in colonial times. The south-eastern Nuba lived in a 'reserved' portion of the Nuba mountains, and were not subject to Christian missionary activities. On independence in 1956, Islamization was encouraged in the Sudan, but the effect, at least initially, was slight.

While Nuba art is socially important from the moment of birth, when the new-born baby is rubbed with oil and red and yellow ochre placed on its head (the decoration being renewed when it is weaned), the designs have nothing to do with their religious beliefs or social structure. For them body painting is not a cosmological art; the body and its celebration is primary, not the symbolism of ritual designs. The use of animal representation has nothing to do with totemism but is chosen because the designs are aesthetically pleasing and appropriate as decorations of the body, preserving balance and a culturally acceptable asymmetry. The great importance of the firm, youthful, attractive body is a reason why decorating ceases when the men grow older and clothing replaces paint. This attitude towards the exposure of the attractive body pervades the whole society, so that men of any age who are sick or injured or incapacitated will wear clothing to cover the body while the illness lasts or the injury heals. This is in strong contrast with the Thompson Indians, among whom old men and women, shamans and chiefs, painted their bodies for ritual reasons, and the injured or diseased body was painted bright red.

The beautiful young Nuban body must be clean, shaved and oiled before it is considered appropriate for decoration and public exposure; if a man has not shaved his beard and his pubic hair he will not decorate. On the whole, however, except at the height of the farming season when time is short, young men are always painted.

Rich deep black is used by the young athletes in the Nuban bracelet fights and it is supposed to make them look bigger and more imposing than their opponents. It is also used when a youth performs praise-song dances, exposing himself, painted, on hearing his praises sung. During this demonstration and dance the men are at the centre of female attention and may be rewarded with a special physical display rite, not dissimilar to the Hagen institution of 'turning head'. A girl chooses a partner and throws her legs over his shoulders in order to show her appreciation of his decoration, his beauty, and perhaps to indicate that she wishes to make a rendezvous with him later.

Among the Nuba the body becomes both the medium and the message. As in many other societies past and present, the human form is seen as the foundation for a work of art—in fact the use of skin and flesh as the artist's medium rather than his inspiration antedated the more conventional categories of plastic arts in the West. In the West, body art has declined to a garish representation of sexuality and vanity. Nuban art, on the other hand, is a fine art, the body being used as a contoured and plastic surface. The body, with its vertical bilateral symmetry and the horizontal arrangement of parts is the most important variable in the style, form and aesthetics of Nuba personal art. Whatever the designs used, the critical factor is their relationship to the canvas-body, which must be complemented and enhanced by colours and patterns.

The Nuban artist knows his canvas well. There are terms for practically all the muscles visible on the body surface and for the depressions between the muscles. Splitting the body in half below the neck, there are over fifty terms in common use, excluding nine for the spine. Many other terms refer to posture and stance, aspects of the body in walking, stepping, prancing, dancing, skipping, and in perspective. The plastic surface of the body, including bumps and scars, may be used in creating the work of art. The shape of the jaw-bone or the curve of the forehead may form part of the overall design. A shoulder muscle may be the bulge of a tortoise shell; the rise of a back muscle the rump of a giraffe; the eyes may become the centre of an elaborate bird's wing. Sometimes the whole body may serve anatomically as the animal being represented, the animal shape being made appropriate to the human form. A man may become a giraffe or a wasp. Wherever possible the anatomical congruence is followed: thus an antelope with stripes over its eyes will be represented by stripes over the artist's eyes.

However, most of the designs are abstract and give the artist more freedom to emphasize the various parts of the body. Non-representational designs may emphasize various features, even rearranging the symmetry of the body to enlarge the eyes and diminish the nose or alter the shape of the head in a pleasing way. Balance is taken into account in a purely aesthetic way, with an eye on the viewers, frequently girls watching the dances, wrestling and ritual races. Colours are used, not symbolically, but to alternate the distribution of light and dark colours on either side of the body. According to Faris, this celebration of the body may be linked with their concern with health, their desire for a strong body. Whatever the case, it is their concern with style and form, using the body as canvas, for aesthetic rather than social or ritual reasons, which makes Nuban art so spectacular and so unusual.

In the West, the gradual acceptance of cosmetics for men is a return to an exceedingly normal situation where both sexes decorate their bodies for a variety of reasons. Curiously enough, there is a connection between the return of Cosmetics for men in the West and Commerce, a link echoed, as we shall see, in certain customs pertaining to the islands east of New Guinea.

In this century, perhaps owing to the austere image brought about by two world wars, men have avoided beauty aids, scents and special hair-dos. It was vaguely thought that a real man should smell of things like tweed and petrol, gin and sweat, tobacco and shoe polish. Yet in the nineteenth century, while cosmetics for women went underground, men used powders and paints and pomades. Napoleon had an expensive and lavish taste in toiletries, and even during campaigns he insisted on a good supply of quality soaps, eau de cologne and almond cream. In the late nineteenth century in America, a standard book on male etiquette advises the use of hair dye, paint, face powder and eye shadow.

Perhaps it was as a result of our own puritanical attitudes towards men's cosmetics that we stressed the decorative display of the male sex in primitive groups and tried to account for it. Darwin, discussing this, stresses that 'in most, but not in all, parts of the world the men are more ornamented than the women and often in a different manner', and attempts an explanation:

> As the women are made by savages to perform the greatest share of the work and as they are not allowed to eat the best kinds of food, so it accords with the characteristic selfishness of man that they should not be allowed to obtain or use the finest ornaments.

Darwin exaggerated the predominance of painting and decoration among men, although the contrast with our society was striking. Now I have already suggested that the apparently obvious explanations of body decoration for men—sexuality and aggression—are not the only ones. In contemporary Western society, advertisers tend to appeal to the warrior, the he-man, in selling cosmetics to men; scents and creams and aftershaves are advertised by boxers, footballers and cricketers. Men are told that the products will make them feel bold, brash, rugged, commanding, vigorous, brisk and stimulating. Sexuality as such is not an important concept in this advertising, partly because men like to believe that they are able to attract women through virtues other than their physical appearance. Moreover, cosmetics for men have to be sold to people who have long believed that paints and scents were only for homosexuals, not for the sexually secure, virile male.

Men are beginning to use cosmetics for the same reasons as women. They want to promote vigorous good health, or the appearance of good health, by artificial means. Men in important and responsible positions are turning to the hair surgeon, the cosmetic surgeon and the make-up specialist, with the idea of looking younger and rested. Older men are sold cosmetics through their fears of retirement, of being usurped at work by younger men, of illness and death. In our culture an ugly, old face cannot be a successful one. A successful man is tall, bronzed, muscular, youthful-looking and has a good head of hair. In other words, men paint for business as well as for sex and war.

This connection between cosmetics and commerce is an interesting one. In my book *Friends and Lovers*, I discussed many cases of bond friendships between people living in different countries, speaking different languages. Friendship was kept alive by the exchange of gifts and trade, and in a surprisingly large number of cases the ornaments traded were ornaments and cosmetics: red ochre, nose ornaments, shell objects. In many cases the efforts trading partners made to exchange an ornament or a cosmetic powder would seem quite out of proportion to the value of the object.

The interplay of social and economic relationships involving ornament and body painting comes out well in the system of exchange known as *kula* found in the islands to the east of New Guinea. In this ring of islands, groups of men take part in an economic and ceremonial exchange, involving the circulation of valuable necklaces and armbands, as well as commercial goods. The partners in this exchange become friends. The closest friends are partners who live in the same village or island, while the overseas friend is seen as an ally, a friendly protector in a strange land where sorcery and other dangers are to be feared. After a long and hazardous sea voyage to visit a foreign country speaking a foreign language, a man's ally, his special *kula* partner, is his guarantee of safety and hospitality.

In New Guinea, the principal exchange involves ornaments; and it is a ceremonial exchange, helped by magic and cosmetics. Melanesians use cosmetics for all social events, as we have seen. The men of the *kula* sail their ocean-going canoes over great distances, and none would dream of embarking without his cosmetic kit. Malinowski calls their unguents and herbs 'magical', though the distinction between the magical paints and perfumes of the South Seas and the pragmatic cosmetics of the urban West is not an obvious one. The *kula* men make 'magic' when a group leaves on an expedition. This is aimed at success in the exchange and is directed at the partner's emotions: it makes him soft, unsteady in mind, eager to hand over to his friend the best *kula* objects.

Arriving at a distant island, where they are not always sure of their reception, the men in their canoes perform further rituals in the form of personal beauty magic to ensure the success of their visit; they attempt to make themselves irresistible to their business friends through the use of spells and cosmetics. They murmur magical formulae, wash in the sea, and rub themselves with medicated leaves and coconut oil. They arrange their hair and draw designs on their faces. Youthfulness and attractiveness is magically applied to the body in the form of scents, dyes and paints. The main aim of the Trobriand businessman is the same as that of the Western businessman or woman: being irresistible, to get the better of the deal. In one of the myths, there is a description of an old and ugly man transformed into a radiant and charming youth through cosmetics and magic. He becomes so beautiful that his business friend is obliged to throw the best ornaments at him.

An ugly old *kula* trader is only too aware that he will not win the prizes without artificial aids; and in the spells associated with cosmetic preparations before the exchange of goods, he prays that he and his partner will become like a pair of parrots, birds which symbolize friendship and love. 'My head is bright, my face flashes, I have acquired a beautiful shape like that of a chief; I have acquired a shape that is good. I am the only one; my renown stands alone.' In Melanesian beauty magic a man's business friend 'hugs him and takes him to his bosom', sits on his knees and takes from his mouth 'the betel-chewing materials'.

Like the Melanesian, the American businessman must consider his clothes, his paunch and his wrinkles. At beauty farms there are 'men's weeks' for executives sent by their firms for beauty treatment in the interests of business. There they receive the same treatment as women 'guests'. Cosmetics in the Trobriand and American cases are magical aids to success in business. The *belief* in the efficacy of the cosmetics and spells makes them effective, since the Melanesian trader or the American businessman believes he is beautiful and young, and the injected self-confidence influences his behaviour.

*chapter two*

# The Tattooed Body

*Sketch of his own moko tattoo drawn by a Maori chief. Maori face tattoos were a kind of personal signature, the owners believing that their personalities were imprinted into these facial marks. When chiefs signed deeds of land sales to Europeans they drew their face patterns instead of signatures.*

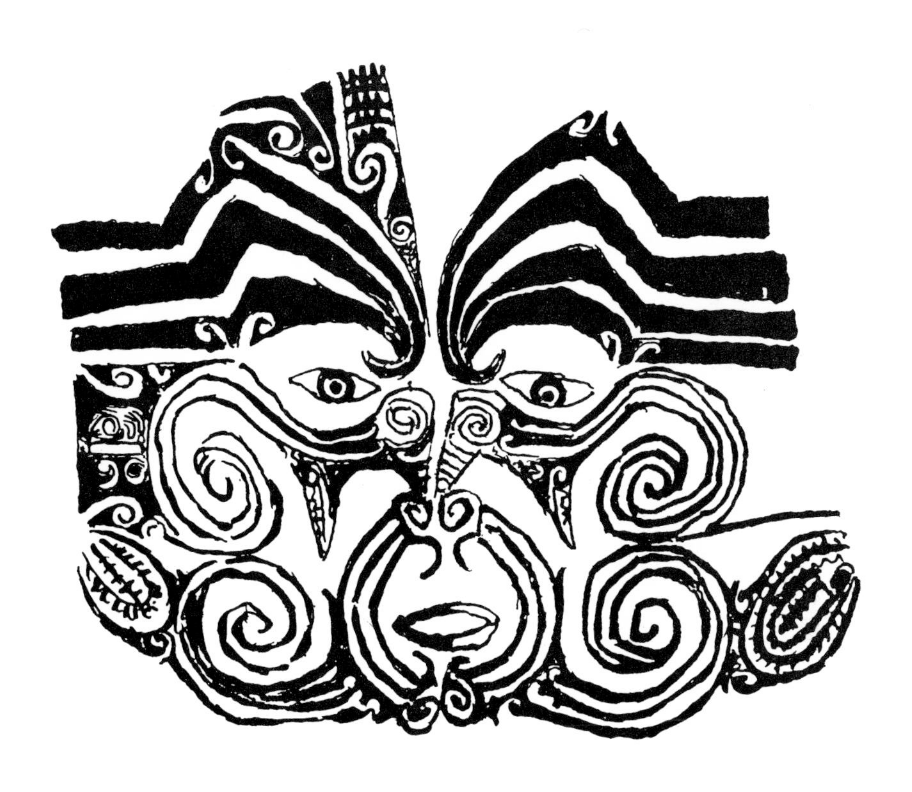

While body painting is an ephemeral art, removable and renewable, tattooing is an indelible, permanent art which cannot be removed without ugly scarring or elaborate over-tattooing. We have examined body painting among the art-conscious Nubans and the individualistic Hageners. Among these societies are no hereditary chiefs or fixed political *status quos*. There is an ideal egalitarianism, and a man may 'come up from nothing' or 'go down to nothing' according to his own personal capacities. But when we consider them in this way we are largely considering the men. Women, in both Nuban and Hagen society, have an overriding *permanent* status as wives and mothers, and in recognition of this they possess permanent body decoration in the form of scarification (Nuba) and tattooing (Hageners).

Hagen women's tattoos are usually confined to the face, and most commonly consist of dots on the forehead arching over the eyebrows, dots under the eyes, or short streaks at the top of the cheeks.

In many parts of the world, but particularly in Melanesia and Africa, the tattooing of nubile girls is not a matter of pure aesthetics but a recognition of their future biological role. At the menarche, a girl becomes a woman who can now marry and have children, and frequently it is the critical parts of her anatomy—breasts and belly—which are decorated. In New Guinea, this work is usually carried out by an older woman; among the Motu from near Port Moresby it begins when the child is small, the hands and arms being tattooed first since they are body parts which are less symbolically important and also less sensitive to pain. At a later stage the belly and chest and back are done. When the girl is considered marriageable, her buttocks and legs and face are tattooed. A feast is given to mark the final stage: the marriageable, permanently marked woman is decked out in finery and parades ceremonially up and down the village. Then for five days she sits on the veranda of the house, displaying herself and her ornaments. During this period she is taboo and may not cook, fetch water or help in the gardens. Among the Roro, the final marks on the breast and back of the neck are made when the girl is betrothed, and on the navel and breast when the marriage is confirmed.

A similar kind of passage rite associated with tattooing is found among the Indonesian people of Borneo. Among the Kajang, the time element in the maturation of the girl is also stressed: a small band or vertical stripe on the finger signifies the 'intention' to complete the final design when she is mature. Among the Kenyah, the girls are tattooed at puberty and then undergo a period of taboo when they are forbidden to bathe in the river. Kajang and Kenyah men may also be tattooed, but in their case maturity is a social maturity which does not arrive automatically. The 'boy' becomes a 'man' when he has proved his powers in battle and acquired social rank through head hunting. A whole hand-tattoo indicates a fully-fledged head hunter; a single tattooed finger shows that he only had a share in the 'kill'.

This pattern of permanently scarring the body as recognition of a permanent change in status is found throughout the world. In the early nineteenth century, a missionary in Paraguay, writing in early nineteenth-century missionary style, recorded:

> At puberty the [Abipoine] girls are tattooed at intervals, meanwhile they are shut up for several days in their father's hut. [Abstinence from meat and fish was enforced but fruit allowed while their chins were tattooed in straight lines.] The Abipoines think that their daughters are ornamented by being thus mangled and at the same time they are instructed and prepared to bear the pains of parturition in the future. Every Abipoine woman has a different pattern on her face. Those that are most painted and pricked you may know to be of high rank and noble birth. If you meet a woman with but three or four black lines on her face you may be quite certain she is either a captive or of low birth. When Christian discipline was firmly established in Abipoine colonies this vile custom was by our efforts abolished and the women now retain their natural appearance.

This smug comment provides a scrap of information on the art of Abipoine tattooing and a good deal on the prejudiced mind of the white outsider.

Europeans first 'discovered' tattooing in the eighteenth century when Cook and other explorers noted its almost universal existence outside their civilized world. But it was a 'rediscovery' rather than a discovery. Tattooing has been known and recorded in Europe and on its fringes since prehistoric times, and the Egyptians have provided direct evidence through their mummies that tattooing was carried out four thousand years ago, particularly on women: dancers, concubines and singers were marked with the symbol of Bes, their divine protector. In 1948 the preserved tattooed body of a Scythian chief was discovered in the Pasyryk mound at Altai. This 2,000-year-old tattoo was preserved by the low temperature of the soil where it was buried and reveals a complex design of animals, birds and fish. Herodotus reports that the Thracians were tattooed: 'To have punctures on their skin is with them a mark of nobility; to be without them is a testimony of mean descent.' According to Pliny, the Ancient Britons stained themselves with a herb and introduced the juice with punctures into the skin so as to form permanent delineations of various animals. 'All the Britons stain themselves with woad which produces a blue colour', wrote Julius Caesar. 'The area is partly occupied by barbarians who bear on their bodies from childhood scars ingeniously formed in the likeness of various animals.' The word 'Briton' may even derive from a Breton word meaning 'painted in various colours'. And just as British sailors relearned the techniques of tattooing in the South Seas and the Far East, Roman legionaries took to the cult of tattooing and it flourished in Rome in the next centuries until the time of Constantine, who declared Christianity the official religion of the Empire (AD325) and forbad face-tattooing on the grounds that it disfigured 'that fashioned in God's image'.

*A finely tattooed dancer from Sarawak, exhibiting the typically regular patterns of the art.* inset *Maori women had fine tattoos around their mouths 'to make them look younger'.*

The art of tattooing barely survived the disapproval of the church in Europe, although the Saxons seem to have been tattooed: the body of Harold was recognized after the battle of Hastings by its distinctive marking, including, it is said, 'Edith' written over his heart like any sailor. However, ornamental tattooing died out in Europe in the Middle Ages and only flourished again after contact with the Far East and the South Seas.

With the opening of Japan to the West in the nineteenth century, and the diffusion of the practice by artists such as Hori Chiyo ('the Shakespeare of tattooing'), who worked on the Duke of York (later George V), his brother the Duke of Clarence and Tsar Nicholas of Russia, the commercial possibilities of tattooing began to be exploited in the West. In 1870, David Purdy, the first English professional tattooist, set up shop in Holloway, London. For a time tattooing had an immense popularity in England—and not only among sailors. It was brought to London's Mayfair by George Burchett, who had learned the art in Japan, and in 1901 many people, including Lady Randolph Churchill, had coronation tattoos done with the royal arms or a patriotic motto. Burchett was practis-

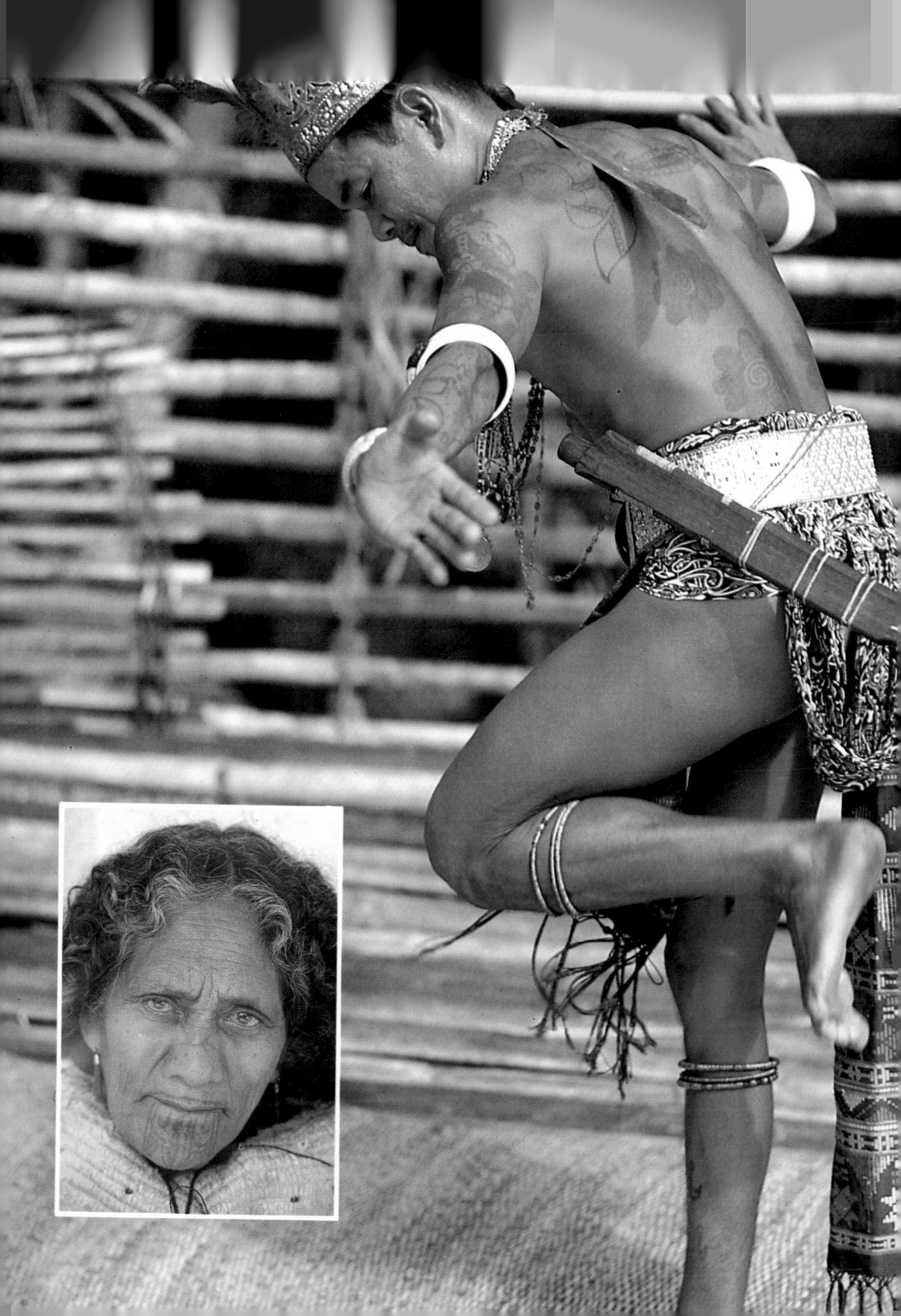

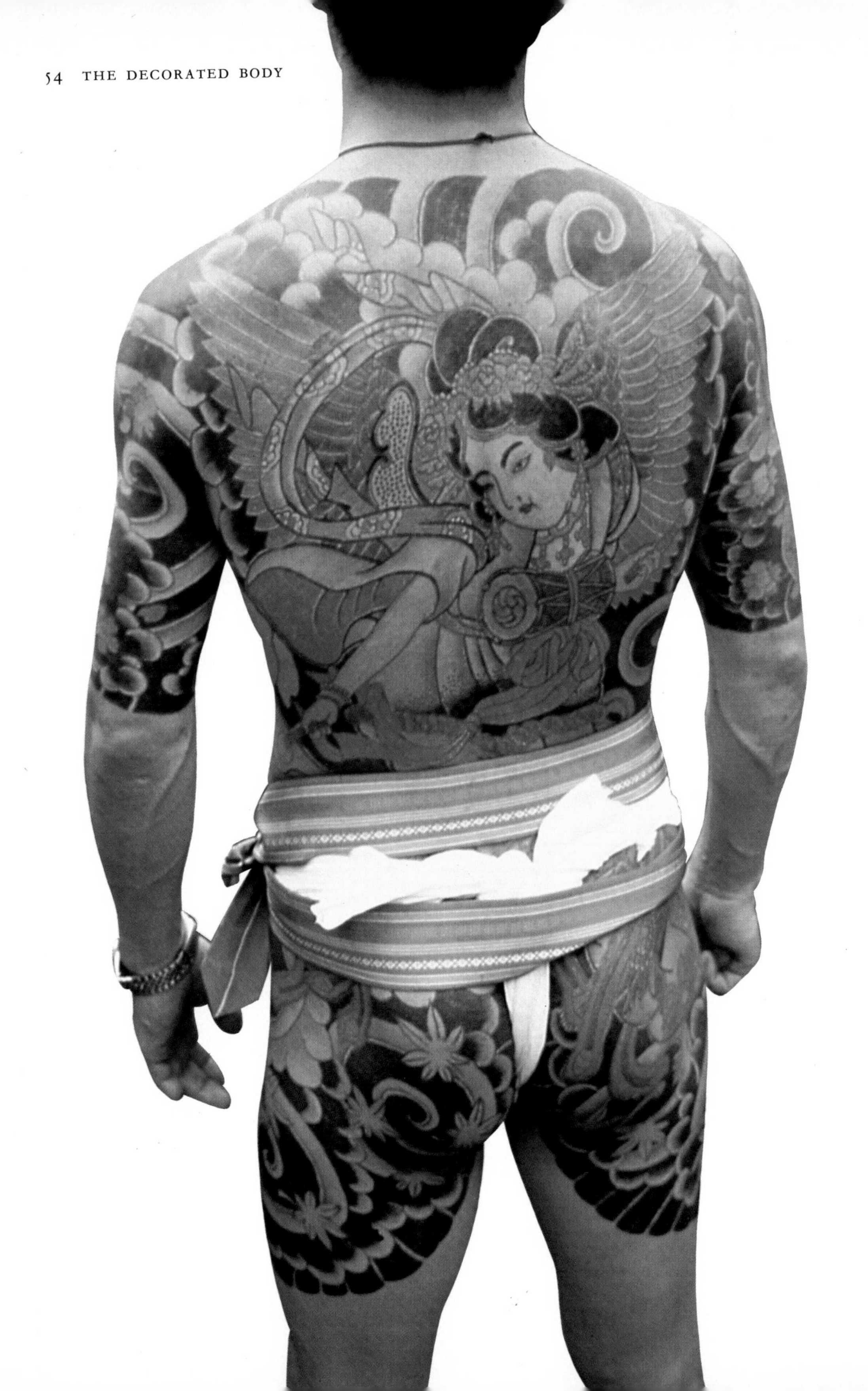

*Japanese tattooing, irezumi, clothes a man. The finished design covers his back, buttocks, upper arms and thighs, leaving the middle of the chest, the stomach and the abdomen undecorated. The cost of one of these magnificent 'suits' runs into thousands of dollars.*

ing at a time, just after the lifting of the long Victorian taboo on face painting, when women were anxious to improve their complexions but were nervous about assuming the gaudy paints of loose women. Electrolysis had been accepted as a method of removing unwanted hair by the upper classes, and as a fresh novelty, while the lower classes took to cosmetics, the upper classes embraced tattooing. Burchett tinted the face by tattooing red lips and dark eyebrows, though the word 'tattoo' was not mentioned.

But while English ladies were permanently tinting their pale complexions, shading their eyes, colouring their lips and having moles and other blemishes removed in the interests of vanity and youthfulness, the great art of Polynesian tattooing was dying fast. Like body painting among the North American Indians, and for the same reasons, tattooing disappeared in much of the Pacific, and the anthropologists who began to appear on the scene towards the end of the nineteenth century were able to record only faded glories on the skins of older warriors and chiefs. A whole body of art had disappeared within a generation of the arrival of Christianity.

Much later, in 1938, the art of tattooing was lost literally 'overnight' on Bellona in the Solomon Islands with the conversion of the whole population to Seventh Day Adventist Christianity. The art of the skin, being on the skin, was there for all to see until the last tattooed person died, but the motivation, the myths, the skills which determined the style and content of the tattoos had been suffocated by the destruction of the social and ritual world. Today tattooing in the Pacific is practised only in certain favoured areas, though Japanese *irezumi* still flourishes.

The techniques of tattooing do not vary much: colouring is pricked into the skin with a needle or sharp instrument. The colouring matter may vary, but apart from the polychrome of Japan and the West, it is usually black—a carbon in some form, such as lamp-black, soot, charcoal or Indian ink.

Among the Kajang of Borneo the tools used were simple and consisted of two or three prickers and an iron striker. The pricker is a wooden rod with a short pointed head projecting at a right angle at one end; to the point of the head is attached a lump of resin in which are embedded three or four short steel needles, their tips alone projecting from the resin. The striker is a short iron rod, half of which is covered with a string lashing. The pigment is a mixture of soot, water and sugar-cane juice, kept in a double shallow cup of wood. The tattoo designs are carved in high relief on blocks of wood which are smeared with the ink and then pressed on the parts to be tattooed. The designs on women are in longitudinal rows or transverse bands and the divisions between the rows marked by zigzag lines. The artist stretches the skin apart with her feet and dipping the pricker into the pigment taps its handle with the striker driving the needle points into the skin at each tap. The operation is painful. Designs are elaborate and beautiful, a mixture of plant and animal designs, anthropomorphic shapes, geometric patterns and abstract forms.

Throughout the Pacific there was a common mode of practice, though there was some variation between the individual islands, which had their own version of the relative mythologies and oral traditions. Unlike the Melanesians of New Guinea, tattooing was practised on both sexes, though the men's tattooing was more elaborate. One of the great Marquesan artists was observed by Melville in the early nineteenth century:

> I beheld a man extended flat upon his back on the ground, and despite the forced composure of his countenance, it was evident that he was suffering agony. His tormentor bent over him, working away for all the world like a stonecutter with mallet and chisel. In one hand he held a short, slender stick, pointed with a shark's tooth, on the upright end of which he tapped with a small hammer-like piece of wood, thus puncturing the skin, and charging it with the colouring matter in which the instrument was dipped. A coconut shell containing this fluid was placed upon the ground. It is prepared by mixing with a vegetable juice the ashes of the 'armor' or candlenut, always preserved for the purpose. Beside the savage, and spread out upon a piece of soiled tappa [bark cloth] were a great number of curious black-looking little implements of bone and wood, used in the various divisions of his art.

Among all the Polynesian peoples tattooing was performed by a professional artist, working with the help of assistants. On Bellona, tattooing was carried out to rhythms, punctuated by the beat of a song, sometimes a steady firm tap, sometimes a rapid succession of tapping. Singing and rhythm helped the tattooed person to fall into a kind of trance which provided relief from the pain. On Bellona, as elsewhere, tattooing was associated with rank and chiefship: the more tattooing a man

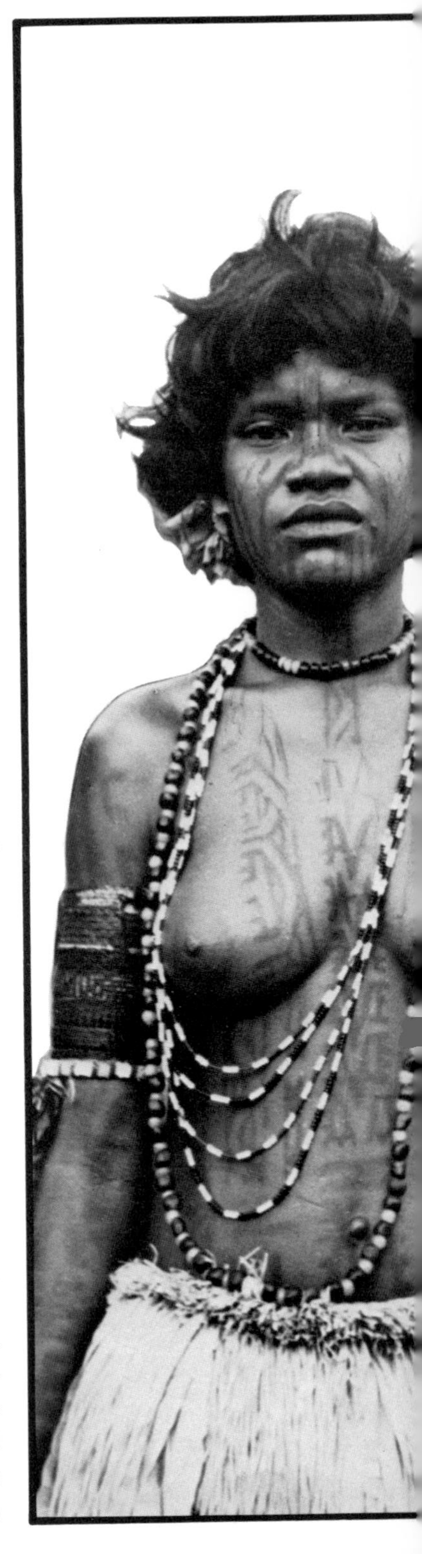

*A tattooed Papuan girl, decked out with twisted armbands and herbs attached to her ears, ready to attend a village dance. The women are tattooed in stages: the final stage is marked by a feast, when the marriageable, permanently marked woman is decked out in finery and parades ceremonially up and down the village.* right *An Iban boy from Borneo being tattooed.* below right *In Borneo the tools for tattooing are simple and consist of two or three prickers and an iron striker.*

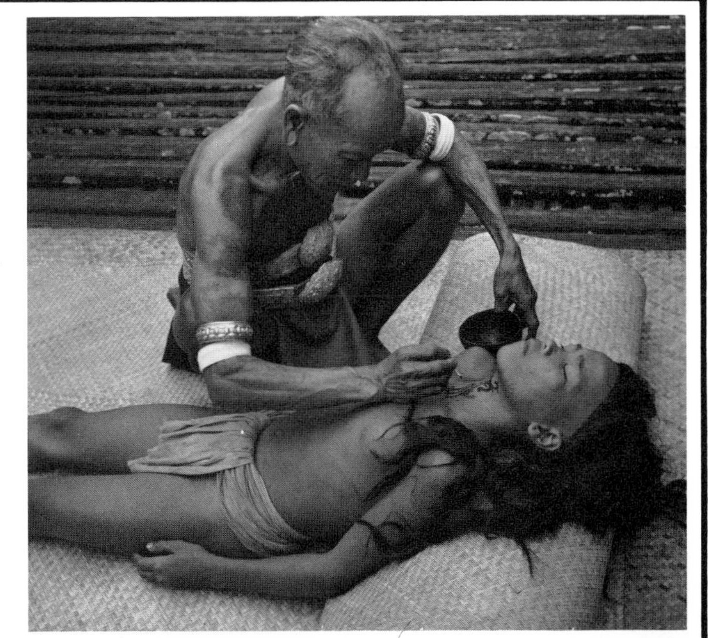

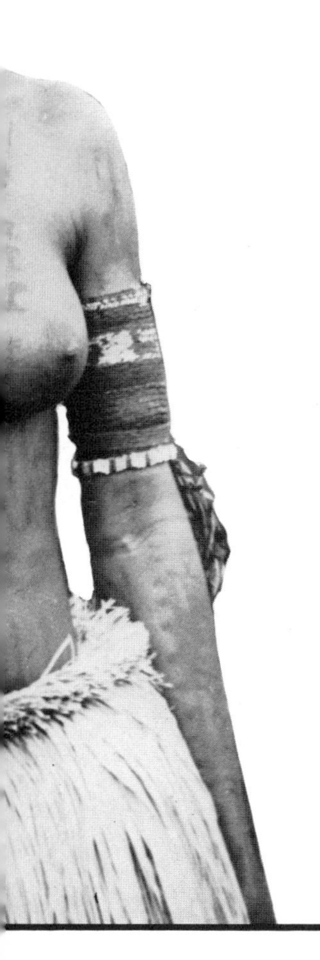

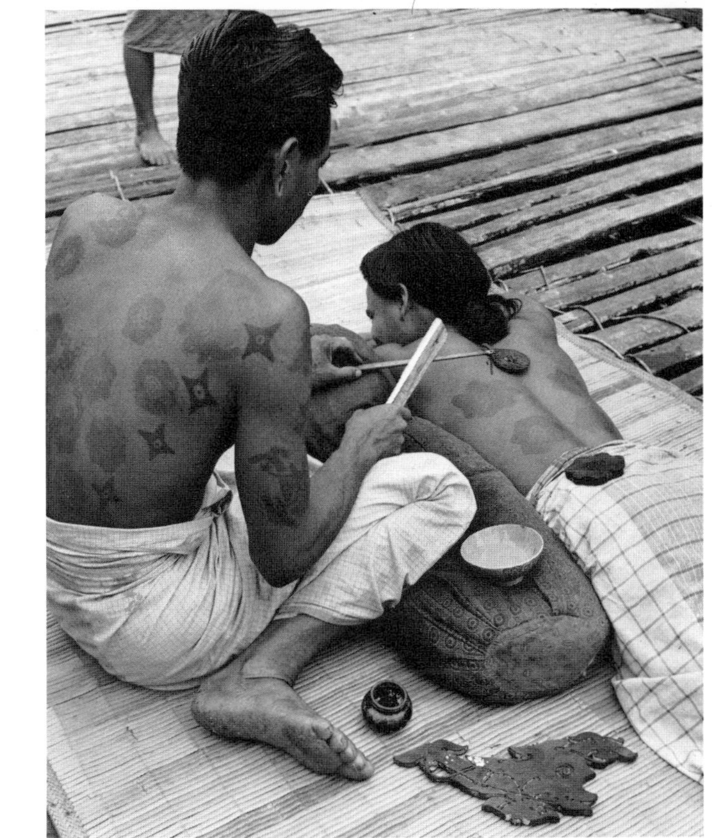

took or was allowed to take, the greater his social standing and the respect he could command. Designs signified social status and in this way social structure governed the style and amount of tattooing. Elder brothers and sisters were allowed the most tattoos: the first-born was allowed eight designs on the back of his legs, but if he had only six, his younger brother was allowed four. The priest-chief had the largest collection of tattoos. He was the only person who could adopt the full design, and his tattooing involved the most elaborate ritual. Lesser priests took other designs.

Certain social occasions also called for tattooing and in Hawaii, for instance, the tips of the tongues of women were tattooed as a sign of mourning on the death of a chief or at any other calamitous event. The artist would immerse the face of the instrument in the colouring matter, place it on the tongue and, giving it a quick sharp stroke with a small rod held in his right hand, puncture the skin, injecting dye at the same time. This became a permanent memorial to the death of a chief, in the same way as Lady Randolph Churchill's tattoo became a permanent memorial to the coronation of Edward VII. Hawaiian women, however, went rather further, and at a royal funeral many disfigured themselves as a sign of grief by knocking out their front teeth and branding their faces with red-hot stones.

I should now like to look in some detail at the technique of New Zealand tattooing, known as *moko*, first observed by Cook and Joseph Banks. It was Cook, indeed, who introduced the word 'tattoo' into the English language as a variation of *tattow, tatau* or *tattaw*, all derived from the Polynesian word for knocking or striking:

> Both sexes paint their bodies, tattow, as it is called in their language. This is done by inlaying the Colour of Black under their skins in such a manner as to be indelible. . . . Their method of Tattowing I shall now describe. The colour they use is lampblack prepared from the Smoak of a kind of Oily nut, used by them instead of candle . . . The bodies and faces are marked with black stains they call amoco—broad spirals on each buttock—the thighs of many were almost entirely black, the faces of the old men are almost covered. By adding to the tattooing they grow old and honourable at the same time . . . The marks in general are spirals drawn with great nicety and even elegance. One

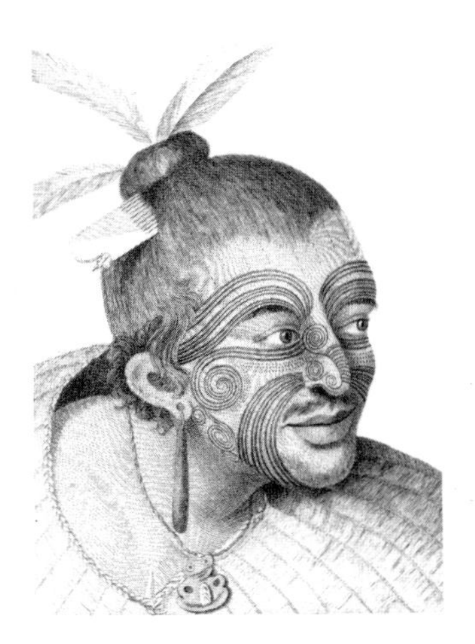

*'The Head of a Chief of New Zealand, the face curiously tataowd, or mark'd, according to their manner.' (From* Journal to the South Seas *by Sydney Parkinson, 1773.)*

> side corresponds with the other. The marks in the body resemble the foliage of old chased ornaments, convolutions of filigree work, but in these they have such a luxury of forms that of a hundred which at first appeared exactly the same, no two were formed alike on close examination.

Neither Cook nor Banks seems to have attempted to understand the motives behind tattooing. In fact they were bemused by the practice. Banks wrote: 'Possibly superstition may have something to do with it; nothing else.' The Europeans, at least initially, saw no beauty in *moko* and no meaning. Even Darwin found *moko* the opposite of beauty and disapproved like a good Victorian:

> The extraordinary manner in which tattooing is here practised, gives a disagreeable expression to the countenances . . . it is moreover probable that the deep incision, by destroying the play of the superficial muscles, gives an air of rigid inflexibility. But besides this there is a twinkling in the eye, which cannot indicate anything but cunning and ferocity.

*Moko,* like all Polynesian tattooing, was a symbol of rank. The great chiefs had their faces and their bodies covered with designs of delicacy and beauty, all free men being permitted the same degree of decoration. Personal, individual designs were made on the face, and it was the ambition of all free men to have a finely tattooed face, which made them conspicuous in war and attractive to women. A face tattoo was also a kind of personal signature, and the Maoris believed that their personalities were imprinted on these facial marks. When the chiefs signed deeds of land sales to Europeans, instead of a signature or a cross, they drew their face patterns, without the aid of mirrors and with great ease. The tattoo also guaranteed fame after death, even if it was the enemy who killed the warriors. Heads of untattooed commoners and slaves were treated with indignity, while those which were conspicuously tattooed were cut off carefully and preserved on a pole. The facial tattoo was also seen as a kind of passport to the next world. After a normal death, the heads of great chiefs were cured over a fire and kept as a memorial of the ancestors.

*Moko* as a technique was unique among Polynesians, since it consisted of a low relief design carved into the skin, with a black pigment rubbed into the cuts. Instead of a needle-like instrument, a chisel was used to make the incisions, driven into the skin with a light mallet. Other instruments were also used, such as one with comb-like teeth fashioned from a seabird's wing bone or piece of hardwood. The finished tattoo was somewhat akin to African scarification. It was rough to the touch since the surface was channelled. As on Bellona, a good deal of ceremony and celebration accompanied the actual tattooing, and in New Zealand the person being tattooed was also subject to taboos: he was forbidden all communication with people not involved in the work. When he ate, he was not allowed to use his hands but was fed by attendants if he were a chief, or lay flat on the ground and ate from a platter with his lips. A man being tattooed could only be touched by the artist and he might not touch his own tattooed head.

*Moko* was a profession, and the tattooer learned his art as a young apprentice, practising on slaves or commoners. To secure the services of an expert tattooer, men showered gifts of guns, canoes, clothes—even slaves—on a renowned artist. Some of a famous artist's work was so highly considered that the corpse was bought and the skin preserved.

When finished, the *moko* face was covered with spiral scrolls, circles and curved lines and no two persons ever looked alike. The lines and curves of the tattoo followed the direction of the natural lines of the face with its depressions and projections, the wrinkles and lines of the forehead, the corners of the eyes and the muscles. The tattoo extended from the throat to the roots of the hair, and before and after the operation every hair that was likely to be in the way was plucked out. On the forehead a series of bars radiated out from a V-shaped centre. The nose had a central ornament with spirals at the bridge and nostrils and another above and on the tip. From the nose to the chin, three or four sets of lines passed the corner of the mouth like a scrolled parenthesis. The upper lip was given various suitable patterns and was scored horizontally, while the cheek and jaw might be decorated with spirals. On the chin, the artist's fancy was given full play and the tracery was more creative.

*Moko* was not only a symbol of rank. It made a Maori chief terrible in war. During battle the constant grimacing and sticking out of the tongue turned the dark lines of the *moko* into a quivering network of aggression. The warrior's aim was to look conspicuous and terrible and so the tattooing was in no sense camouflage.

Slaves and commoners only received minor tattoos, while the women were tattooed around the mouth and on each side of the nose, on the chin, in the space between the eyes, and a little on the forehead and the back part of the legs from heel to calf.

If Polynesian tattooing was an art, Europeans, with their nervous approach to the permanent body arts and used to the designs of their own crude tattoos, have found it difficult to accept. Yet the Maoris decorated their bodies with inspired genius. Their tattooing was central to their whole aesthetic outlook and to their appreciation of the beautiful body. It was closely associated with their sexual attitudes and their relationship to the natural and supernatural world. After the initial shock of seeing a naked tattooed body, some objective Europeans did begin to recognize the artistry of the *moko* tattooers. Even Banks wrote: 'It is impossible to avoid admiring the immense Elegance and Justness of the figures in which it is form'd, which in the face is always different spirals, upon the body generally different figures resembling something of the foliage of old Chasing upon gold or silver; all these finished with a masterly taste and execution.'

Other visitors remarked on the balance of the designs: the minute accuracy of detail, the spiral basis of the ornamentation so well adapted to the curvilineal shape of the human body. Buttock designs, for example, involved a precise spiral line with the starting point at the centre of the most fleshy part, the line successively coiling out like a watchspring to cover the whole area. With the sure hand of a master, difficult geometric forms, parabolic curves, involutes of circles and Ionic involutes were imprinted in the skin. There was never any trace of confusion in the design. The artist had as clear a conception of the finished design as a European fresco painter.

Levi-Strauss has pointed out the strong resemblances between *moko* and the facial decorations of the Caduveo of South America: 'complexity of design, involving hatching, meanders and spirals . . . the same tendency to fill the entire surface of the face, and the same localization of the design around the lips in the simpler types.' And these analogies exist despite the fact that one art is tattoo and the other paint, one rigidly symmetrical *(moko)* and the other asymmetrical.

Other superb examples of the art of Polynesian tattooing are found on the Marquesan Islands and in Samoa. The latter is less well known because of the extreme reticence of those who practise tattooing and because the most elaborate markings are covered with the traditional loincloth. For the most part, Samoan tattooing uses a symmetrical arrangement of lines, dots and crosses on the backs of the hands to form zigzags and rhomboids, and at the back of each knee, where the operation is extremely painful, a finely pointed star is placed. The oblong, lozenge, triangle and V-shaped marks are used in multiple combinations. The inner frontal aspect of the thighs shows a remarkable series of lines of the 'frigate-bird' pattern which gradually converge as they approach the groin. One design which is peculiar to Samoa is a kind of ornamental fishhook armed with numerous barbs. A common pattern found in Polynesian designs is like the crown of a palm tree, springing from the central line of the back and gracefully curving around both sides. In Tahiti, Darwin noted that the body of a man ornamented in this way was like a noble tree embraced by a delicate creeper.

Tattooing of comparable beauty, skill and complexity, while very different in appearance, is to be found in Japanese *irezumi*, where the body is transformed from a naked being into a masterpiece after months of work by a consummate artist working with an awl and gouge on a canvas of flesh. This great Japanese art is now in decline, but fine examples can still be seen on men working on building sites, in public baths and on beaches.

Japanese tattooing has had a long and chequered history. It was first ascribed to the peoples of Kyushu by the Chinese chronicle *The Records of Wei*:

> Men great and small all tattoo their faces and decorate their bodies with designs . . . They are fond of diving in the water to get fish and shells and originally decorated their bodies in order to keep away large fish and waterfowl.

The early primitive designs indicated differences of rank. Later they became purely ornamental. *Irezumi* flourished in the seventeenth and eighteenth centuries when even great artists like Utamaro designed tattoos. During this period merchants, as opposed to the nobility, were not permitted to wear fine silks, brocades, or gold and silver ornaments. They could however wear an expensive secret tattoo. So while a rich merchant wore the appropriate plain kimono vividly embroidered on the *inside* with gold, his son might wear an expensive tattoo on his arm or thigh.

Later there was a reaction against tattooing when it became

right and below right *Japanese tattooing, irezumi, is a fine art. The designs are dictated by the curves of the human body. An appearance of solidity is given to scenes and figures by close attention to perspective, background and choice of colours. Among the places where irezumi can most commonly be seen today are building sites and public baths.*
below *Tattooing in the Marquesan Islands was also a fine art. This intricately and symmetrically tattooed Marquesan is illustrated in* The Races of Mankind *by Robert Brown, 1873.*

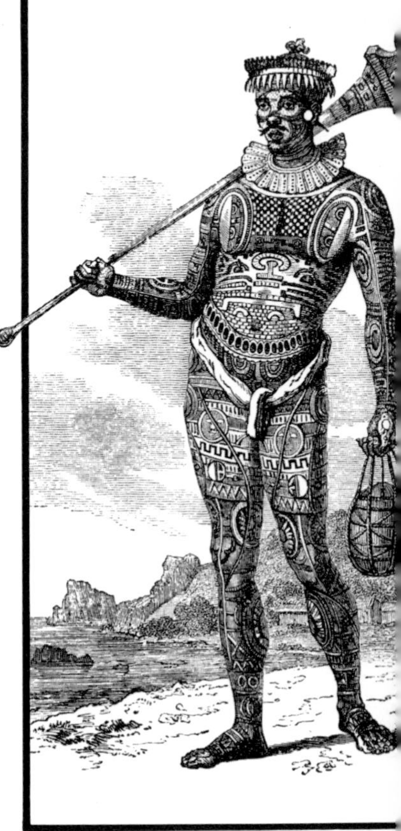

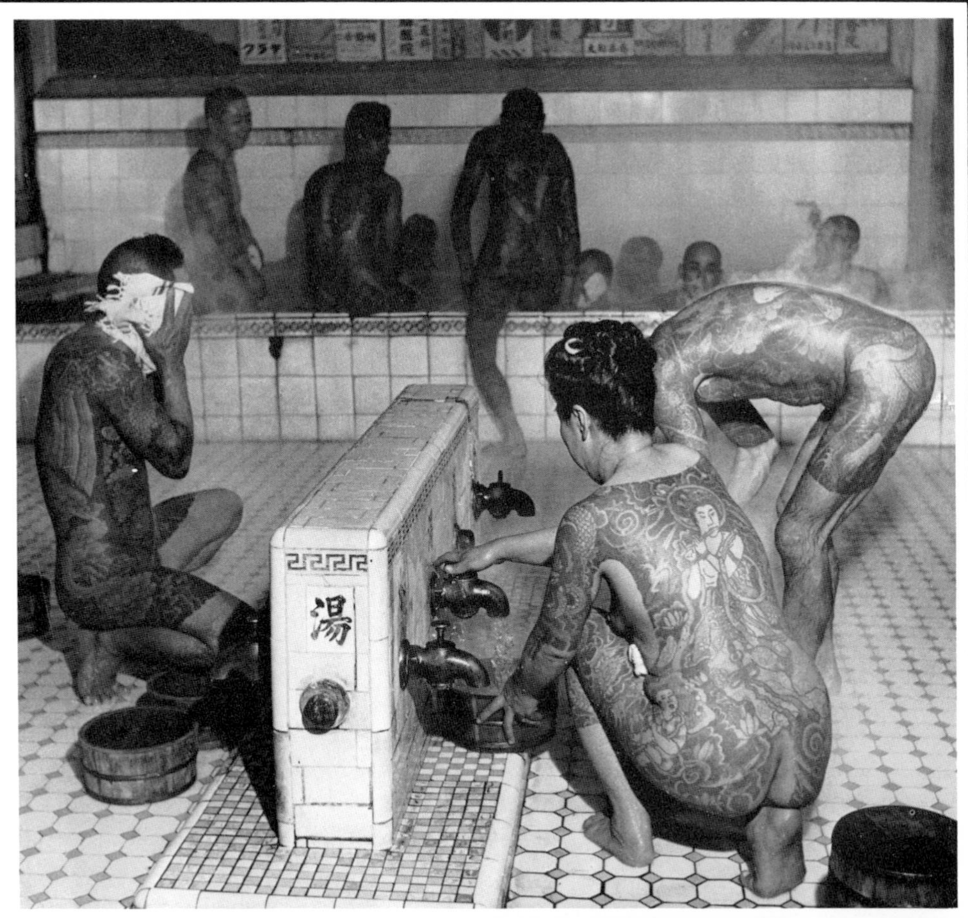
湯

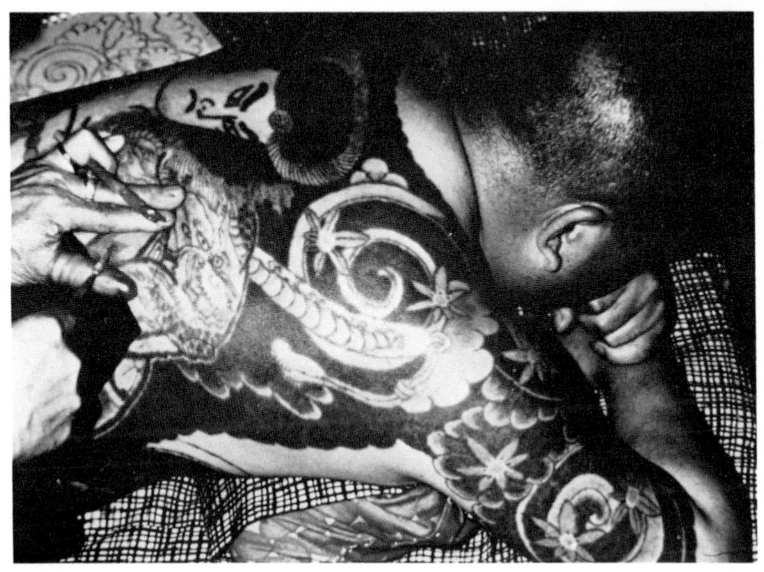

confined to the lower and criminal classes. At one stage it became little more than an instrument of punishment. The criminal was marked on his forehead and around the eyes so that proof of his crime was visible to all—and the result was ostracism. In the nineteenth and twentieth centuries tattooing was associated also with certain groups: fishmongers, gangsters and gamblers; or it was used as a kind of imitation clothing by the poor. Geishas, on the other hand, were often tattooed with remarkable finesse, usually on the back, and somehow classical Japanese tattooing has survived and earned a well-deserved reputation as a fine art. It is an art which has grown out of a long tradition and developed its own distinctive style.

*In Japan, irezumi has its own art galleries and private museums devoted to the display of fine skins. Enthusiasts even bought the skin off a man's back, making a down payment and collecting the skin at his death. The skin on the wall is a prized specimen belonging to Tokyo University Museum, and taken from the body of its 80-year-old owner.*

In Japan, *irezumi* has its own art gallery, a private museum devoted to the display of fine skins; enthusiasts would buy the skin off a man's back, as admirers of *moko* bought a Maori's head. They made a down-payment and collected the skin when the man died.

The Japanese use tattooing to give personality to the naked body. A nude to them has never been considered 'divine' or even beautiful as it has in the West. Like Caduveo painting, tattooing removes the vaguely animal element from the human body. 'Unfortunately horrible is the sight of the naked body. It really does not have the slightest charm.' So erotic drawings never depict naked people and erotic women are never nude. A man or woman tattooed by the *irezumi* artist is never defencelessly nude without clothes. In fact tattooing 'clothes' a Japanese. The finished design covers the back, the buttocks, both arms to the elbow and the upper thigh, leaving the middle of the chest, the stomach and the abdomen undecorated. Even the bare skin, incorporated into the overall design, acquires an appearance of artificiality. With a completely tattooed suit of clothes, a fireman or a builder could simply put on a loincloth and be considered well dressed.

This 'suit' is very expensive, as befits a work of art. A full suit, if the artist is a well known master, can cost thousands of dollars, and those workmen, carpenters, rickshawmen and concubines who undergo the painful, lengthy business can usually afford little else.

The artist works with a variety of colours, taking more than a year to finish a whole body tattoo. First the design is selected, usually from a collection of traditional patterns in a chapbook. The design is drawn on the skin in black ink. The dye is then applied. Following the outlines, the artist uses a series of

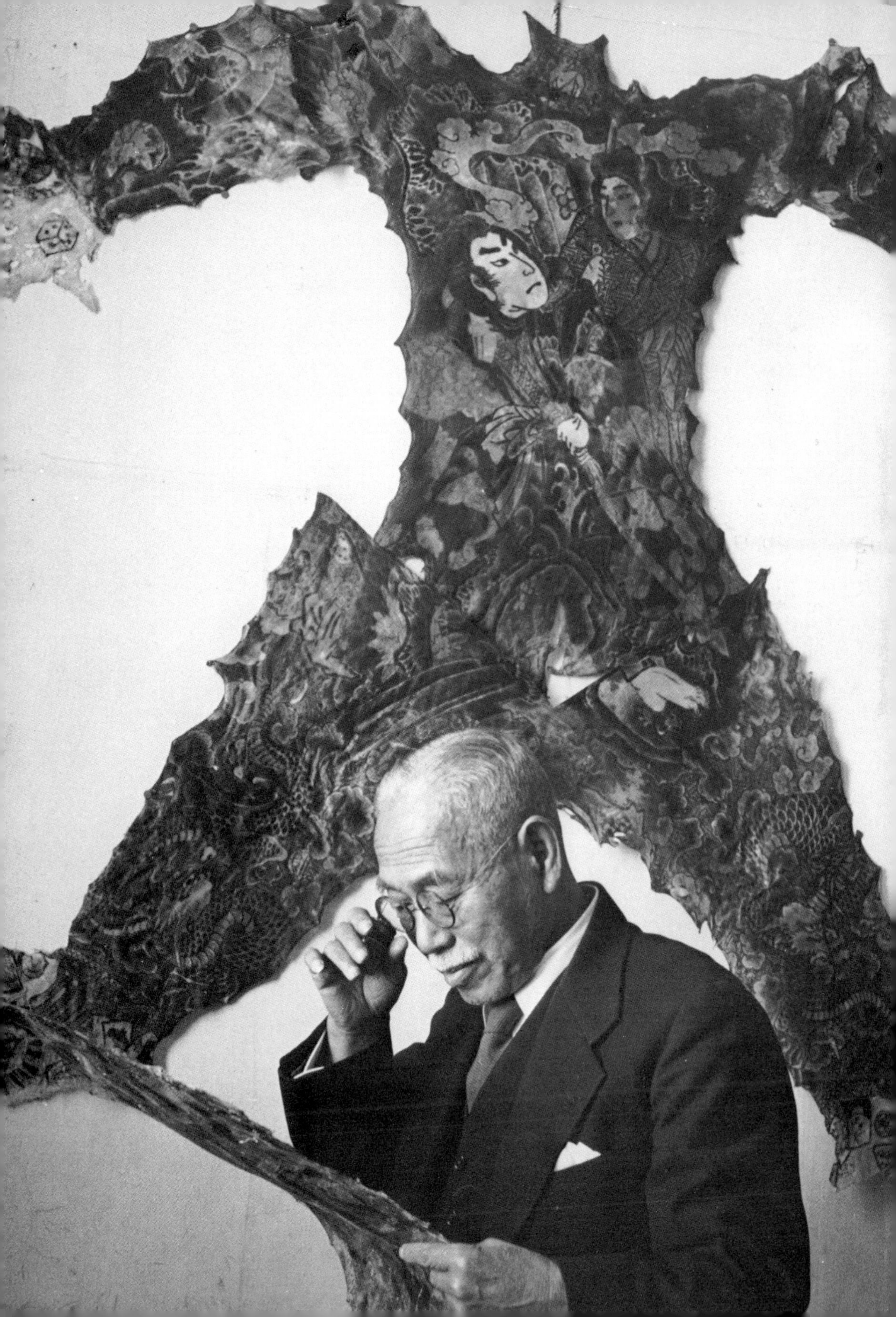

triangle-shaped gouges and chisels. The brush, full of dye, is kept steady by the little finger of the left hand, while the gouge is held in the right, rubbed against the brush and pushed up under the skin. When a thick clear line has been achieved, the artist, using the full traditional range of colours, works the design into the skin. The visits last for several hours, or as long as the client can endure the pain.

The designs are traditional, and include the dragon, giver of strength and sagacity, the carp, folk heroes, Chinese sages and Japanese deities. There are landscapes, floral designs, famous lovers, young men and snakes. The distinctive style is based on the work of several great artists, such as Hokusai and Kuniyoshi, working in the eighteenth and nineteenth centuries.

The palette is that of the Edo period. The main tint is black, which turns blue under Japanese skin. Green is also used, together with a light blue and a beautiful red which, however, is so painful that only a few square inches can be applied. Some of the work in *irezumi* is microscopic. Vermilion is used for bringing out the details. Backgrounds are a bluish grey which may vary in intensity so that a piebald effect is produced. Only Japanese tattooers have been able to master the values of light and shade employed so effectively in the piebald areas. In a deeper blue or red, birds, flowers, faces and demons appear.

Professional *irezumi* artists, after their long and arduous training, produce spectacular results. An appearance of solidity, notably lacking in European tattooing, is given to scenery and human and animal figures by close attention to the laws of perspective and choice of background. The form of the design is dictated by the curves of the human body, the curvilinear technique resembling the forms of Polynesian tattooing and the curls and whorls of Art Nouveau. Moreover, the motion of the lines and figures on the living skin is taken into consideration, and on the moving muscles of a tattooed Japanese you can see a tree blowing in the wind, a fish swimming slowly with a lazy lash of its tail, the graceful swoop of a bird on the wing.

Japanese tattooing is an undisputed art with a fine sense of overall design comparable to the work of the Maoris and Marquesans. It has a strong and unified style and is an art which exists for itself, art for art's sake with a primarily decorative purpose.

I have deferred a discussion of the much clumsier tattooing in the West to the chapter on the Social Body.

*A romanticized sixteenth-century view of a tattooed Pictish woman, by Theodore de Bry after John White. According to Julius Caesar the ancient Britons were tattooed with animal patterns, and it is possible that the word 'Briton' is derived from a Breton word meaning 'painted in various colours'.*

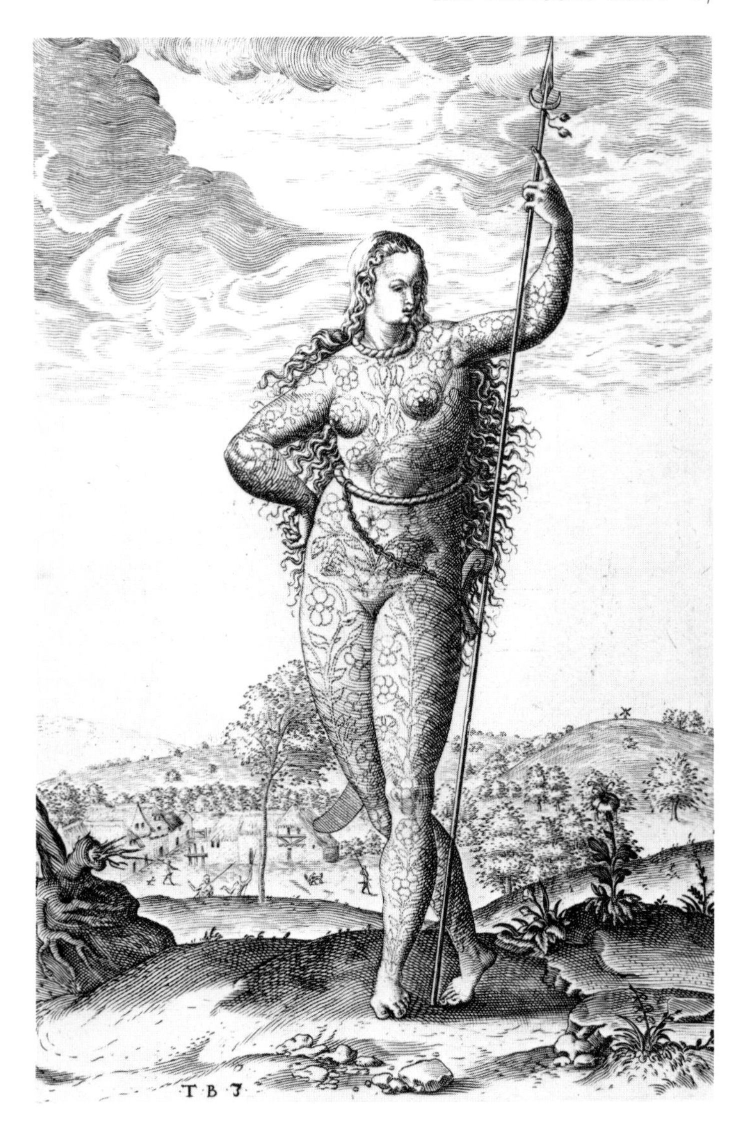

*chapter three*

# The Scarred Body

*A German statesman, whose individual valour was indicated by the scars of physical ordeals in a way very similar to the North American Plains Indians. University students slashed their faces during duels, pouring wine into the wounds to provoke exaggerated scarring as proof of their strength and manliness.*

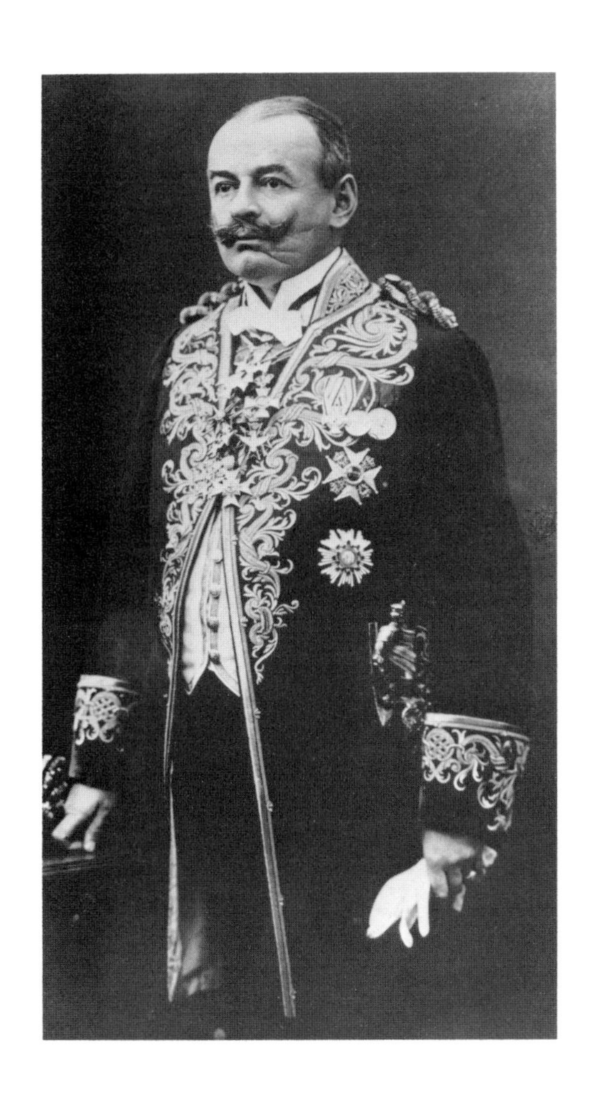

THE TECHNIQUE of pricking and dyeing (tattooing) is mirrored in some parts of the world by the more drastic operation of cutting and raising scars, known as scarification or cicatrization. Scarification is common in Africa, since tattooing is not effective on dark pigmented skins, and the resulting scars vary from rough, ugly keloids to complex and delicate patterns, which are as much fine examples of body art as Japanese *irezumi* or Caduveo painting. Scarification, perhaps more than any other body art, tends to indicate social status and social structure, emphasizing the continuity and way of life of a particular tribal group or class. It nearly always, however, follows aesthetic as well as social canons.

*Scarification varies from large raised keloids to complex and delicate patterns; whatever their aesthetic appeal, these prominent scars hold deep symbolic meanings for the people concerned. Here a bead of raised keloids decorates the brows of a Shilluk from the Sudan.*

In New Guinea, as we have seen, girls are tattooed at puberty. In Africa, Nuba girls, from southern Sudan, undergo a series of scarifications which is also related very closely to their physiological development. The first of this series of marks is a pattern of scars cut on either side of the abdomen, joining at the navel and continuing to a point between the breasts. At puberty, when the breasts begin to fill out, the girls are taken by older women to the mountainside, where they remain in isolation until the scars heal. A second set of cuts is made at a girl's first menstruation and consists of a series of parallel rows under the breasts which is continued round to the back and over the whole torso. After the weaning of the first child, a final scarring takes place, and the woman is marked all over the back, the neck, the back of the arms, the buttocks and the back of the legs to the knee.

The scarification operation is performed with two instruments: a hooked thorn to lift the skin and pull it up, and a small blade with which the raised skin is sliced to produce a protruding scar. The more the skin is pulled up before cutting, the higher the resulting keloid. A high keloid lasts longer and is considered more attractive.

Among many African people, including the Nuba, both boys and girls are scarred on the face after puberty, and this scarring is repeated a few years later. The primary intention of African scarification appears to be to enhance the individual's beauty, though the Nuba maintain that cuts above the eyes aid sight, and those on the temples are said to relieve headaches.

Scarification, like tattooing, is disappearing, having been highly disapproved of by missionaries and banned by colonial governments. In contemporary Africa, 'tribal marks' have been outlawed by such governments as the Ivory Coast as manifestations of 'anti-patriotic tribalism and primitive sur-

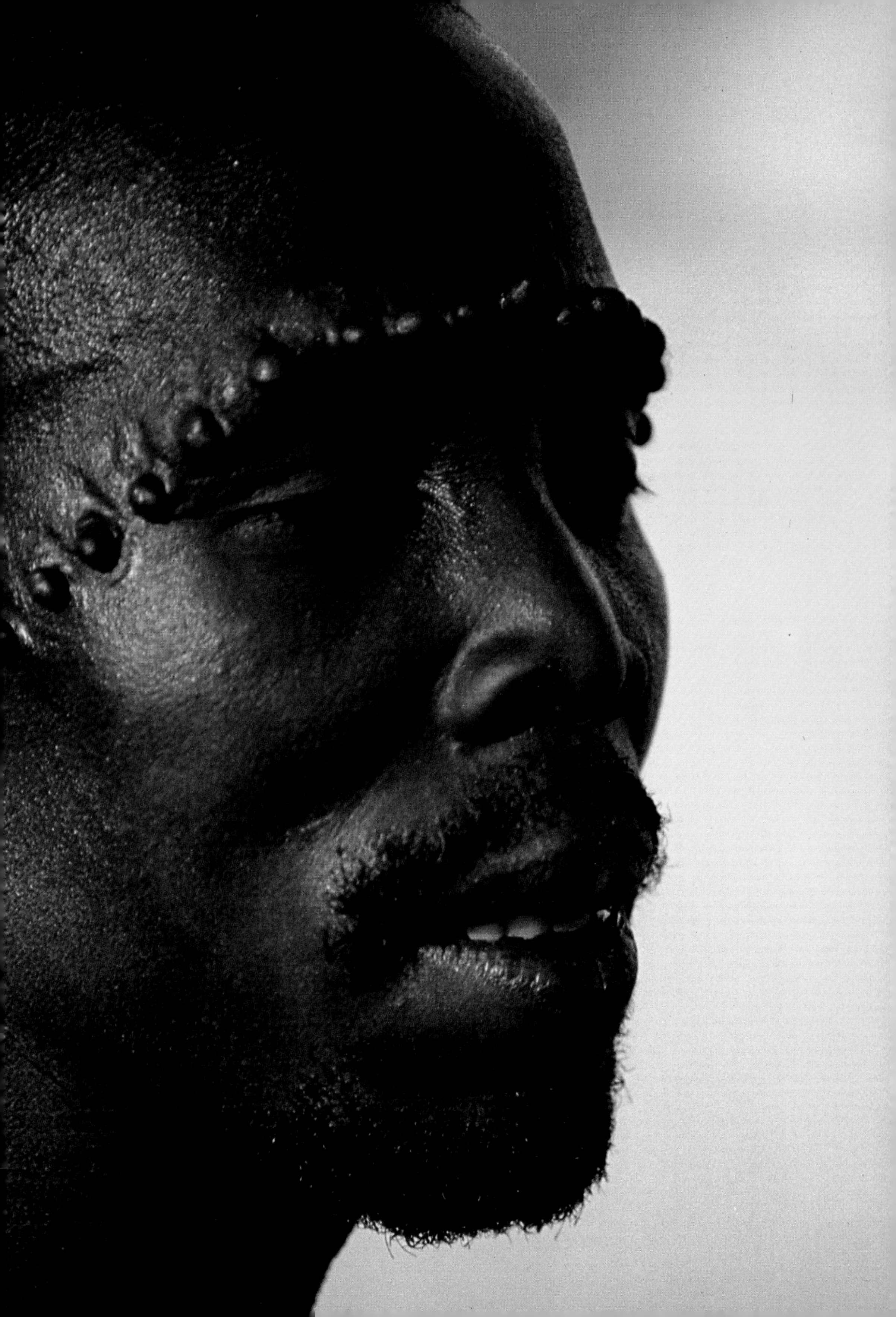

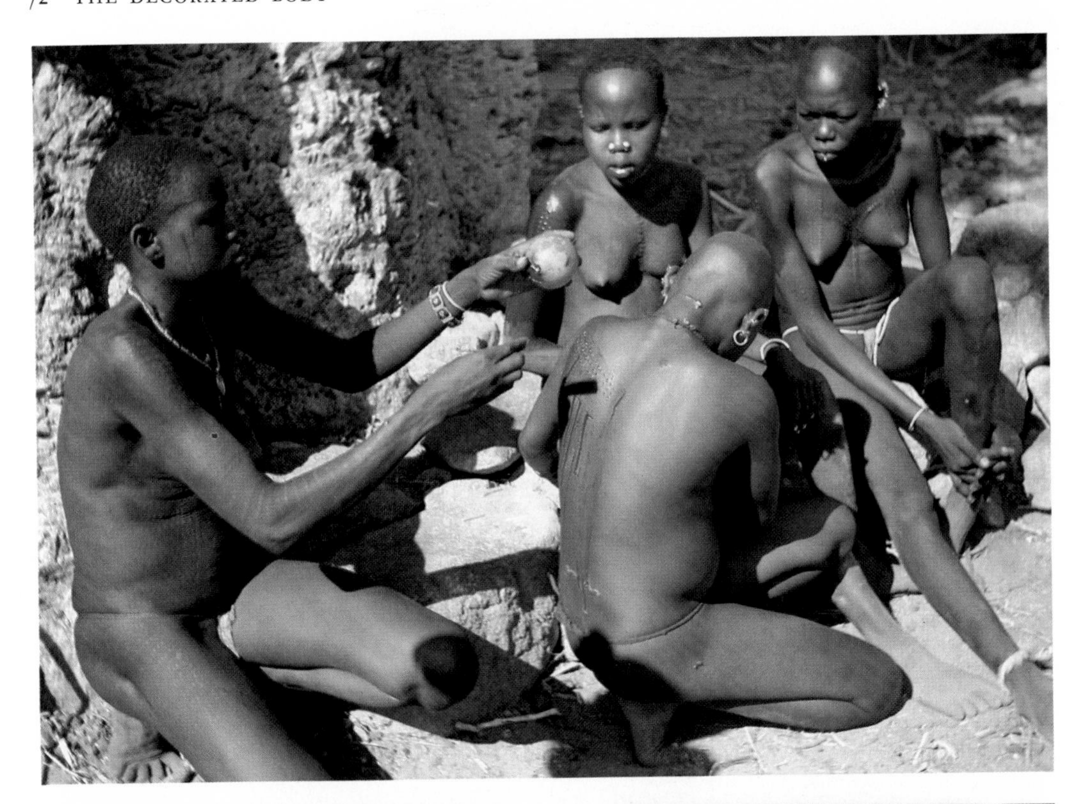

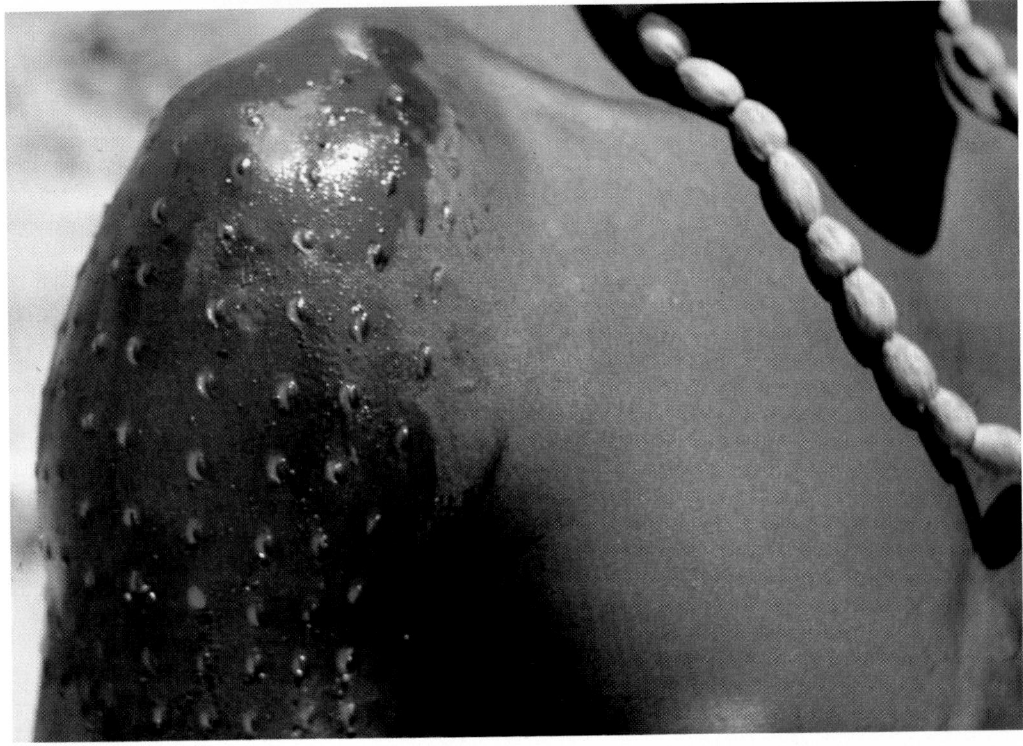

*This Nuba girl will be both beautified and marked socially through the scarification she is undergoing.*
below *Fresh scarification wounds, produced by lifting the skin up with a hooked thorn and slicing the raised skin with a small blade, creating the protruding scar.*

vival'. I suspect that few readers will doubt the wisdom of these governments or be able to accept that scarring is an aid to beauty. On the whole, Westerners regard self-mutilation as a sign of psychopathology and have always taken a poor view of its manifestation in both our own and exotic societies. Perhaps it would be as well to have a closer look at our own practices and attitudes to scarification, which like tattooing and body painting is not unknown in Western society.

A man with a scar or a strong, damaged face may often be judged more attractive than one with unmarked features. Scars reflect masculinity, and give a man a martial, virile air, and some people induce them to this end. Like the North American Plains Indians, among whom individual valour was indicated by the scars of physical ordeals, war or the marks of self-inflicted wounds, Western criminals and gang members sometimes induce scars. Extreme members of modern Punk Groups mutilate their bodies in this way and are adjudged confused and primitive. Yet German university students slashed their faces *in der Mensur* (students' duel) and poured wine into the wounds to provoke exaggerated scarring—evidence of their strength and manliness. Even among American football heroes scars are sported as proud adornments. A wound that does not fester and leave a deep scar is not considered worthwhile, and impostors have been known to slash themselves with a razor and rub salt into the wounds to give the impression that they too bear the fine disfigurements of honour. Psychologists may dub such actions as those of confused minds, yet they quite happily send older middle-class patients with confused minds to surgeons for plastic skin therapy. Where is the difference?

In Africa, however, scarification has more serious purposes. Even on African carving the marks are often reproduced with great care since they indicate the precise status and identity of the person portrayed in a mask or portrait statue. Tribal marks are usually cut on the face and may be 'hollow' or 'raised' according to the treatment of the wounds. The open-style flat scars which are not raised by colorants or irritants allow the best work, and are found among the Bateke, where facial scarification follows the lines and structure of the face and is as delicately wrought as Maori *moko*. These fine sweeping lines are repeated on Teke masks. The 'raised' method, which uses scarification to make the welts and lumps known as keloids, allows a greater variety. It can also produce beautiful patterns, although some techniques result in ugly

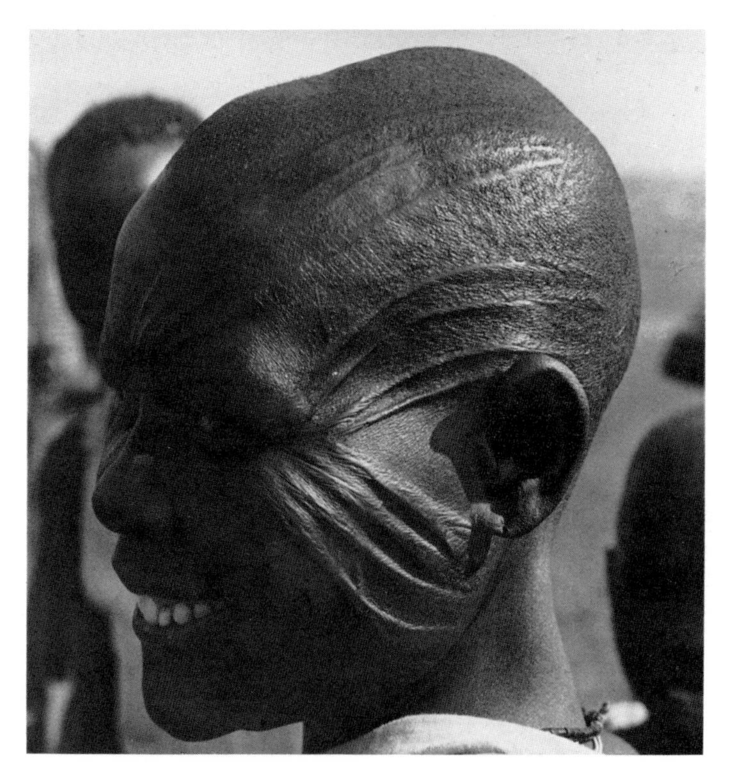

*Scarification is common in Africa, since tattooing is not effective on dark skin. It tends to indicate social status but it always follows aesthetic as well as social canons. The scarification on this Dinka woman from the Sudan clearly follows the lines of her skull and cheekbones.*

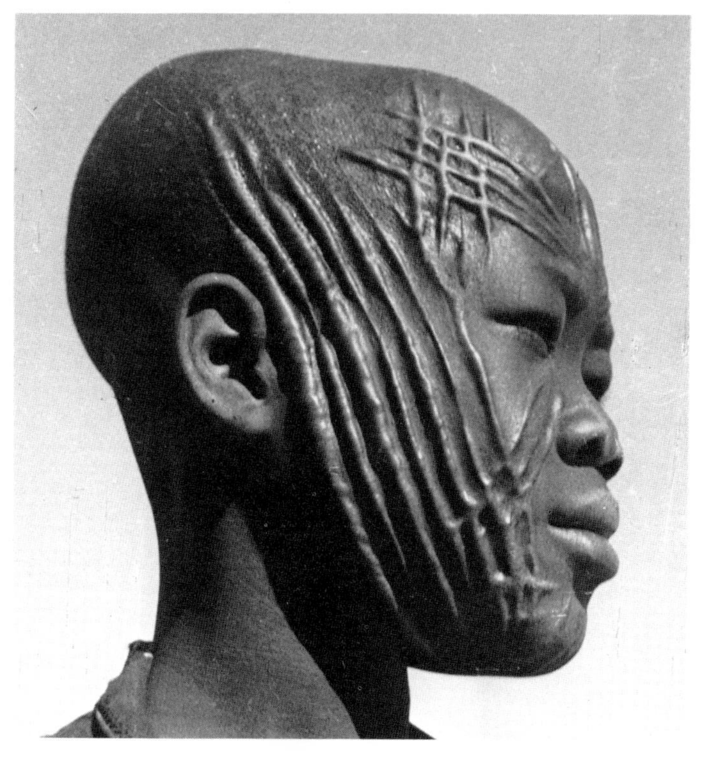

*'Tribal marks' have been outlawed by many African governments. Scarification not only serves as a tribal mark, however; it also plays a large part in initiation rites, when proof of an initiate's fitness, endurance and manliness is required, as is the case with this young man from Chad.*

protuberances as big as tumours.

Among the Bangwa of Cameroon (and the Bamilieke) scarification was practised not to distinguish tribes but as an indication of individual status (such as royalty) and a mark of personal beauty. By the time I was living among the Bangwa in the 1960s the practice had died, though I saw a few fine examples of the art. Women, who prior to the 1940s and 1950s wore no clothes at all, were traditionally marked as a sign of their status—as married, fertile women are among the Nuba. They were cut by experts on the chest and the stomach before marriage; and after the birth of their first child they were scarified on the back, mainly in a complex design of solar or lunar disks. Men, usually chiefs or members of the royal family, were marked in a similar way, the designs including many of the motifs found on their elaborately sculpted house-poles and other sculpture. At the same time scarification was used as preventive medicine: a four-pointed star on the right side near the liver was supposed to preserve a man from hepatitic infection; in the case of sickness caused through spirit possession, cuts were made all over the body to free the person from the influence, rather like blood-letting or cupping in Western society.

Blood-letting, of course, is a major factor in the differences between the temporary body arts (painting) and the permanent (tattooing and scarification), and it is accompanied by pain. *(Il faut souffrir pour être beau.)* For this reason, as we shall see in the chapter on Passage Rites, tattooing and scarification are ideal for marking important status changes where at critical moments of life, such as puberty, the necessity for courage plays a large part in operations which demand proof of the initiate's fitness and endurance. And along with the pain there is the blood. Some societies stress the importance of the piercing of the skin and the drawing of blood, the blood carrying away imperfections or the evil contained in the body. (The Nuba girls are scarified in isolation on the mountainside above the village because the blood is considered evil and polluting.)

Sylvia Plath in a short story about tattooing suggests that pain and blood are part and parcel of the 'ceremony' of tattooing even in our own society. 'The sailor is gone from behind his eyes now, off somewhere in Tibet, Uganda or Barbados, oceans and continents away from the blood drops Carmey is drawing in the shadow of the eagle's wings.'

The Tiv, a large population who live in the Benue Valley of

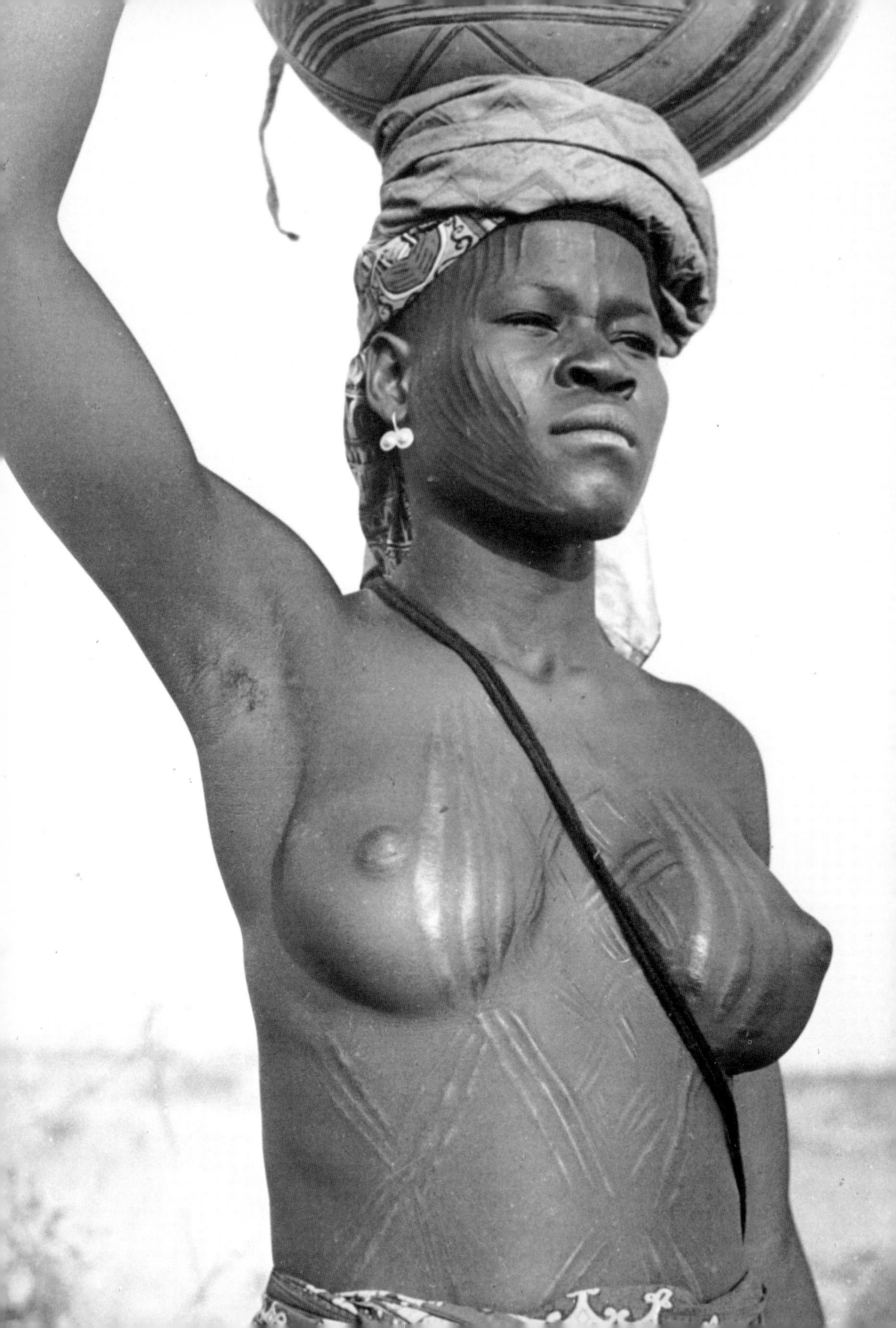

*In the Cameroon, women were traditionally marked by scarification as an indication of their status as married or marriageable women.*

Nigeria, told the American anthropologist Paul Bohannan that suffering plays a necessary part in becoming beautiful when they scarify their bodies and chip their teeth. Asked if the cutting had been painful, a man who had undergone scarification for purely aesthetic reasons replied: 'Of course it is painful. What girl would look at a man if his scars had not cost him pain?' Scarification is a prized decoration paid for in pain, and the beauty of the work depends on the amount of agony experienced.

Scarification among the Tiv is an art which is intimately involved with their particular ideas about physical beauty and their general aesthetic concepts. A beautiful Tiv woman is well-dressed, with a smooth, oiled, fine-coloured skin, chipped teeth and an incised skin surface. The skin is improved by being rubbed with oils coloured with camwood and henna. Apart from scarification, the women also make facial marks using the twig of a certain tree which leaves a spot if pricked into the skin, the spot disappearing after two or three months. These temporary tattoos are white and very attractive on their black skins. They are also used to outline the design for permanent scarification.

While most of Tiv scarification is aesthetic and does not reflect social status, the designs may serve to mark the bearer's generation, since the patterns change every ten years or so according to current fashion. Fashion is particularly important for the men, women stressing their preference for young, handsome men with new patterns. The various forms of cicatrization include a type of flat shiny scar, which is usually made along the arms and down the back, lumpy marks made by the hook method described for the Nuba, and another kind of scarring made by a nail. Each of these methods of cutting is followed by the use of a styptic agent to stop the bleeding, and the application of ashes, charcoal or indigo to make the scars more prominent.

The decorative face markings may change the Tiv features in a remarkable way. Nail marks, for example, which are very deep, dramatically affect the fall of the shadows on the face, prominent cheeks being made more prominent by the double of the shadows cast on them. A nose can be made longer or shorter by the use of a deep mark.

Most of the scarification designs are common to both sexes and consist of geometrical patterns or representations of birds, animals and fish. Bohannan says that all these marks have a purely cosmetic purpose, though he agrees that the markings appear to be made at special times during a person's life. (One woman had saved an empty space on her forehead for the time she would leave her second husband!) However, like the Bangwa and the Nuba women, and like the tattooed girls in Melanesia and Indonesia, the Tiv have a special marking incised on a woman's belly. These designs, centred on the umbilicus, are the most characteristic of the Tiv scars and are not subject to the whims of individual fancy or fashion. They are called 'catfish' by the Tiv, a word which in the Tiv language is very similar to the word for 'lust', and it is a favourite joke among the men that the design of the tail of the fish is sometimes represented by a knot of scar between the breasts. The design has a long 'neck', and 'fins' which are represented by the wing-like extensions of the designs on both sides of the navel.

Paul Bohannan sensibly describes Tiv scarification from the point of view of the Tiv themselves; and the Tiv see them as beauty marks, nothing more. However, the aesthetic is only one point of view. It would not be far-fetched, for example, to suggest that the designs on the women's bellies are symbolic of the girls' biological roles as wives and mothers. The Tiv themselves, when confronted with this suggestion, agreed that the scars might be connected with fertility. They said that the scars are tender for some years after they are made and these artificial erogenous zones make women sexier and hence more fertile. Other facts indicate that there may be deeper meanings.

A Tiv girl is scarified when she becomes nubile. The operation is performed with the girl lying arched over a stool. The design, which no Tiv man could ever wear, is drawn in charcoal before it is cut. The lines are cut with a razor and the dots by the hook method. Charcoal is then rubbed into the wounds. It would seem likely that the designs made on the girl's belly at this critical period must be linked with Tiv notions of fertility and religion. The meanings can be sought by comparing them with the sacred objects they represent. The Tiv have a notion of magical forces or emblems which safeguard the welfare of the community and individuals. The most important of these emblems is a brass pipe known as the *imborivungu*, which is used in rites to promote the fertility of women and the land. Women are in some ways similar to the sacred pipe and are themselves considered sacred, because of their role in reproduction, and women are peculiarly sacred at puberty, when they become capable of producing life. Puberty

*The patterns on the skins of Australian Aborigines are produced by cauterization or by cutting the skin with a sharp object and rubbing in ashes or clay to accentuate the scarring. This young woman is from North-western Australia.*

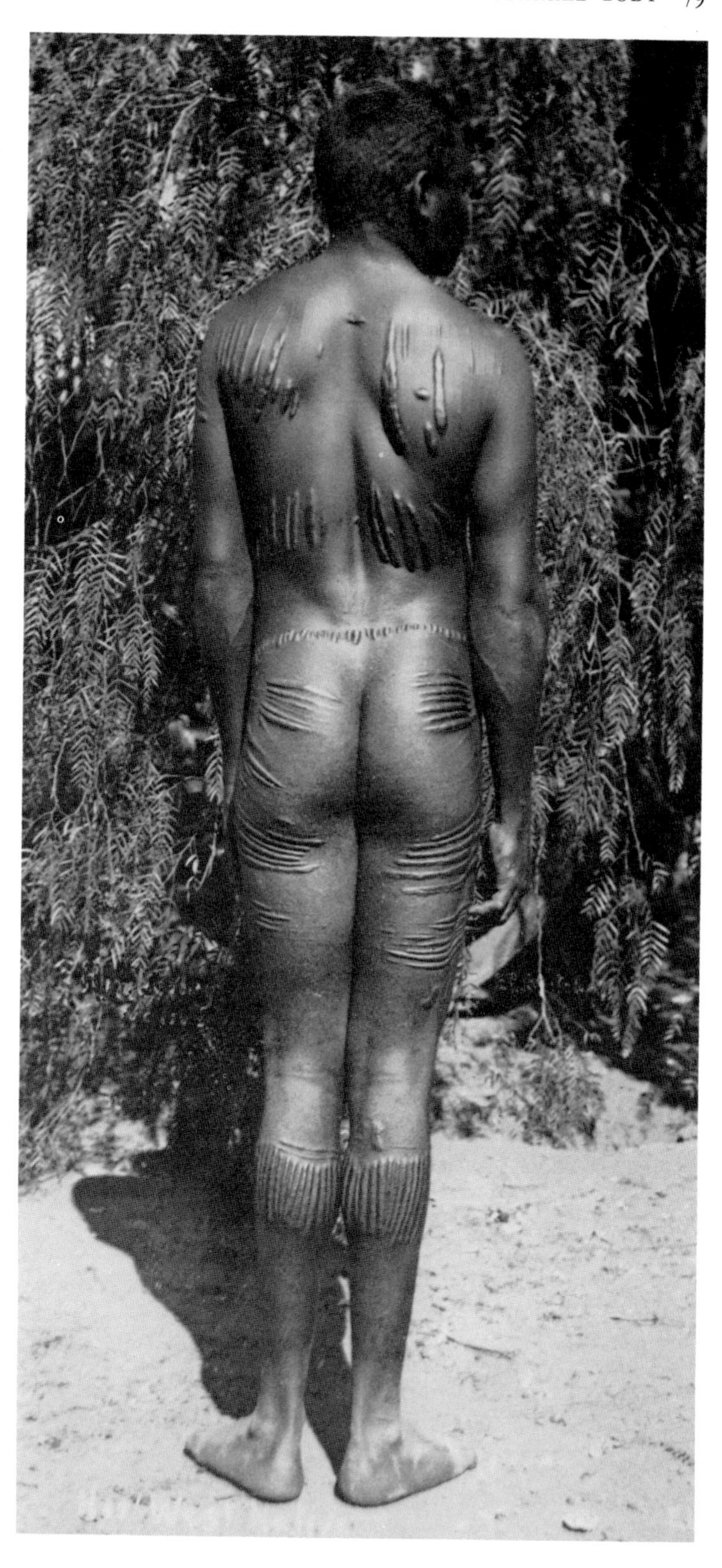

is the time when a girl's belly is scarified and she is transformed into a sacred object.

Another anthropologist, Bruce Lincoln, believes that the patterns on Tiv women's bellies are not representations of a fish with a clitoris-tail, as Bohannan would have it, but a symbolic representation of a line of living persons and of ancestors —a tracing on the skin from the past to the present. The circle at the navel represents the living community based on age-sets and generation differences which are symbolized by the rippling of the concentric circles out from the centre and into the future.

The scarification of a woman's belly is therefore a *rite de passage* and a symbolic representation.

I have stepped gingerly into the deep waters of the symbolic meaning of body art in order to make the point that the patterns involved, which may seem haphazard or merely 'pretty' to an outsider, have a deeper conscious meaning for the people concerned. Too often I have noted the shocked expression of a European confronted for the first time with the deep scars of an African's tribal marks. I was born and brought up in Australia and gained the general impression that the Black Australians were a simple-minded folk who treated their bodies with contempt, gashing and burning the skin as an idle pastime. Australians certainly do mark their bodies, but not 'just for fun'. Sometimes there may be no formal meaning attached to the weals which they raise on their skins in patterns which can be intricate and decorative: they need not indicate clan or tribal membership and do not always have as elaborate a symbolism as their body painting. As among the Tiv, the patterns may depend on personal taste. They make a series of horizontal weals across the chest, abdomen and back, with vertical marks on the upper arms. The marks are produced by cauterization—the application of a glowing stick—or by cutting the skin with a piece of flint and rubbing in ashes or clay to accentuate the scarring. As well as these decorative marks, the Australians are also 'mutilated' with the scars of self-inflicted wounds made on the occasion of mourning ceremonies. Men's thighs and arms may also be scarred with wounds inflicted during a duel. Women sometimes wound themselves at funerals by jabbing their skin with a digging stick, or if a child has died they may amputate a finger joint.

And at this point we have left the realm of aesthetic scarification and entered that of mutilation which, while containing elements of cosmetic transformation, usually has a deeper meaning.

*chapter four*

# The Mutilated Body

*Human bodies are rarely left in their 'natural' state. Until very recently in the West, the worst kind of body mutilation was imposed on women in the name of Fashion: the constriction of the waist and chest by tight lacing, which resulted in the deformation of the body and its internal organs and often led to pulmonary diseases. This cartoon depicts 'A correct view of the new machine for winding up the ladies'.*

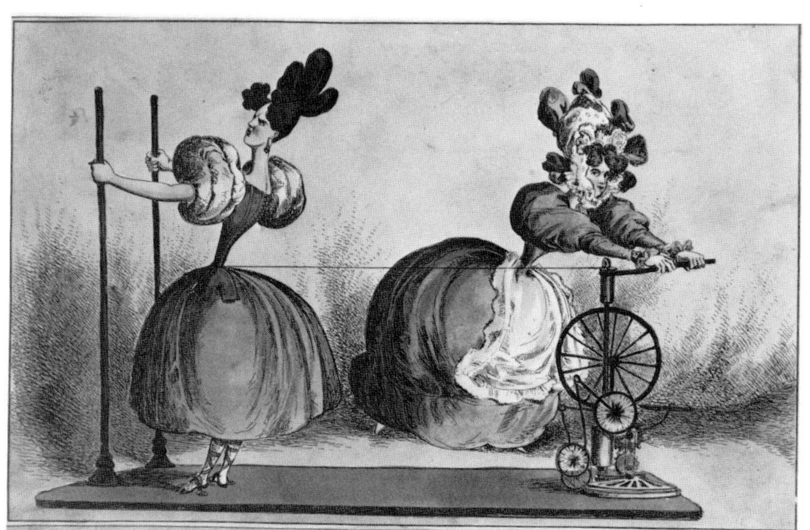

A CORRECT VIEW OF THE NEW MACHINE FOR WINDING UP THE LADIES

DARWIN SAID that Man admires and exaggerates what Nature gives him. However, Man not only exaggerates—he deliberately deforms the body out of all recognition, often enduring exquisite agonies as he twists and compresses, amputates, swells and shrinks, pierces and bruises and otherwise torments the natural shape of the human form.

In the West, mutilation is mostly confined to cosmetic surgery, although foot, waist, chest and skull deformation have been practised in the past largely through a crushing desire to conform to stereotyped but ever-changing body ideals. In many other societies mutilation has a less frivolous basis, and involves religious beliefs; but even in the West, blood-letting, flailing and scourging and other sado-masochistic attacks on the body have been associated with Christian devotion and penitence.

Among the Ancient Mexicans, religious fanatics also held that to attack the flesh was meritorious in the eyes of the gods. Certain Aztec priests practised abscission or entire discerption of the male parts. In Yucatán they let blood from their bodies, cutting their ears all round and leaving them so as a sign of penitence. On other occasions they celebrated their gods by piercing their cheeks or underlips, cutting off parts of the body, perforating their tongues laterally or cutting loose flesh from the pudenda and leaving it as 'ears'.

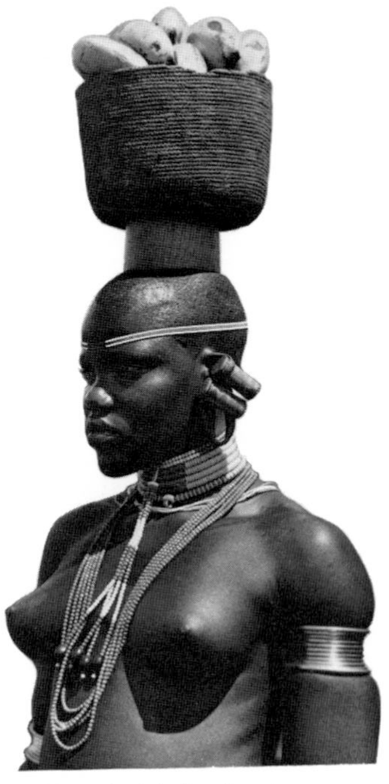

*A Butende girl whose bangles were placed on her arms and legs when she was young. Their restriction causes the arms and legs to bulge alarmingly, as she puts on more weight, but their tightness appears to cause no harmful effect.*

In the West we still pierce our ears, straighten our noses, and deform waists and chests by corsets. Our purpose would seem to be to draw attention to certain parts of the body. Western women have commonly accentuated the mouth with a slash of red, the ears with earrings and the eyes with black, blue or green make-up. Other peoples wear ear-plugs, labrets, lip-plugs, nose rings, penis sheaths or penis rings. I only want here to insist that the propensity to deform or alter the natural shape of the body is a universal one.

No distinction can, therefore, be made between civilized and primitive practices. Europeans deform the waist and foot; Africans mutilate the genitals; Australians lop a finger in mourning; a fashion-conscious Western woman lops a toe to squeeze into her pointed shoes. Among the Caribs, young girls wore two-inch broad bands of cotton wound around the ankle and just below the knee. The bands were never removed, so that the calf muscles swelled to an abnormal degree between them, while the parts of the legs which remained bandaged were hardly thicker than the actual bone. The Incas kept their children wrapped in swaddling clothes for three

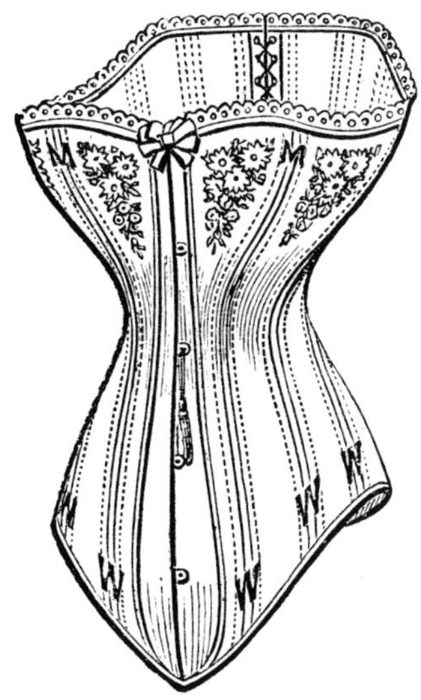

*Corset, to create the ideal female shape in 1888.*

months, believing that if they released the arms and legs before that time they would grow feeble. Similar ideas were held in Europe until recently; people believed that the limbs and orifices of the child were sensitive points which were protected by swaddling from mystical attack.

In Europe until very modern times the worst kind of body mutilation was imposed on women in the name of fashion—this was the constriction of the waist and chest by tight-lacing, which resulted in a deformation of the body and its internal organs, often leading to pulmonary disease and constituting a gratuitous attack on the body unequalled anywhere in the world. (Only in Crete can we find other examples of the violently constricted waist, and there it seems to have been attained by the wearing of a rigid girdle from childhood.)

Corsetry in Europe was introduced in the fifteenth and sixteenth centuries. At first the bodies were simply tightly bandaged, but later the bandages were reinforced by small boards about two inches wide with strings attached for tight-lacing. As well as this positively sadistic attempt to alter the natural contours of the waist and abdomen, the women were also constrained to place lead plates on their breasts to make them flat-chested, so that it became practically impossible to nurse babies. The deformation of the body was so severe that women fainted if the constrictions were removed and were even forced to keep the apparatus on in bed. Botticelli's women, with their prominent abdomens, owed their shape to tight-lacing.

In the nineteenth century, tight-lacing became as primitive a mutilation as clitoridectomy. Shortly after birth, a leather belt was tied firmly around the baby's waist. When the child's growth snapped the stitches, the belt was replaced by a second, equally tightly sewn. These constrictions gave a disproportionate width to a woman's hips and shoulders, and this became the ideal female form. When the girl married, it was her spouse's privilege to remove the final belt, which he cut off with his dagger on the marriage night.

Despite the damage we willingly inflict on our own bodies, it is still very hard to write objectively about some customs in other societies. Female circumcision is one example. We may feel shocked at the idea of clitoridectomy, yet we show little reaction when we mutilate our own bodies in the interests of vanity and youthfulness. A woman who has learned to be ashamed of her full breasts undergoes an operation as unpleasant and as primitive as the excision of the clitoris. In order to diminish the size of large breasts, incisions are made around the base of the breast and up to the nipple. Since the nipples would be displaced and pulled down under the breast as a result of this 'aesthetic surgery', the nipples are cut out and stitched to a higher position. Naturally the breast loses its functions; its sensitivity and scars remain. This operation, unlike clitoridectomy, is an operation made in response to fashion and in the interests of conformity, not in response to tradition, religious belief and social commitment.

Clitoridectomy is a custom reported by Strabo from Ancient Egyptian times. It is still practised by certain pagan and Moslem peoples from India to Morocco. The Nubians (not to be confused with the Nuba), who inhabit a strip of the Nile between Aswan, Egypt and Dungola Sudan, perform ritual operations on very young girls, excising the clitoris and closing the vulva with scar tissue. This type of operation is known as Pharaonic or Sudanese excision and is actually an infibulation. Before the rite, the girl—the small 'bride'—is adorned with gold and dressed in new clothes. In the manner of a real bride her eyes are made up with kohl and her hands and feet dyed with henna. The operation is quickly performed by a midwife who excises the labia minora, part of the labia majora and the clitoris. The women present chant, 'Now you are a woman!' 'You have become a bride!' 'Bring her a penis, she is ready for intercourse!', punctuated by cries of joy and Koranic incantations. Raw egg and green henna are applied to the wounded parts and the child's legs are tied together, sometimes for as much as forty days. The healing process generally provides the scar tissue for the complete closure of the vulva, except for a small urination orifice, which is kept open by a match or a reed tube. Throughout the healing period she is treated as a bride or a woman who has given birth.

The explanation given by the women themselves for this brutal operation varies. Almost invariably, the immediate answer is that the excision is a religious obligation. Nubians believe that it symbolically purifies the child, promoting cleanliness and fertility. Of course, the closing of the vulva, like the ring put through the foreskin of a boy in medieval Europe, prevents sexual contact; in the Nubian case, it also ensures perpetual virginity and so obviates the possibility of a shameful pregnancy.

Such explanations are direct expressions of the belief that women have an inherently wanton character which is physiologically centred on the clitoris. However, modern women in

Nubia still insist on the excision of the clitoris. One of their main reasons is that the operation is an aesthetic one: without the operation the female sexual organs are disgusting both to the eye and to the touch. Unexcised women are considered unclean, unattractive and somehow beastly. It is a serious insult to call a man 'son-of-an-uncut-mother'. There is a clear feeling, as with all mutilations and cosmetic surgery, that unless it is done the person remains disfigured and ugly. Moslem women shave their pubic hair just before marriage and, with the clitoris removed, the vaginal opening does have a clean-cut and simplified look. On the whole, however, the operation must be associated with the Moslem belief that women are weak, passive creatures incapable of controlling their sexual urges.

Among other peoples the reasoning is more mystical. The Dogon of Mali consider children who have not had their foreskin or clitoris removed to be physically and spiritually androgynous. For the girl, the clitoris is a symbolic male, a makeshift with which she cannot reproduce and which also prevents her mating with a man. She has it removed, since anyone trying to mate with an unexcised woman would be frustrated by opposition from an organ claiming to be his equal. Similarly, when a Dogon boy is circumcised and his foreskin, his makeshift female half, is transformed into a lizard, he attains his full masculinity.

Circumcision is performed far more commonly than clitoridectomy. Except among the people of the Middle East and Ethiopia the operation is performed at puberty. The methods are various. Among some groups of Brazilian Indians an artificial circumcision is produced by pulling the prepuce back and tying it securely behind the glans. Circumcision among Jews is a religious act establishing a covenant between the Lord and his people. In the United States in the 1930s and 1940s, whatever its subterranean symbolic meaning, circumcision was fashionable and almost *de rigueur*, and justified on hygienic grounds. In parts of Australia, as well as undergoing circumcision at puberty, an operation known as subincision was performed later in adolescence when the urethra was split open from its normal aperture back towards the scrotum.

It is perhaps no mystery that the penis has always been a centrepiece for body decoration, an object for ritual as well as aesthetic attention. The Dayaks pierced the penis and inserted objects into the foreskin. In societies where the penis is not mutilated, attention may be called to it by such devices as

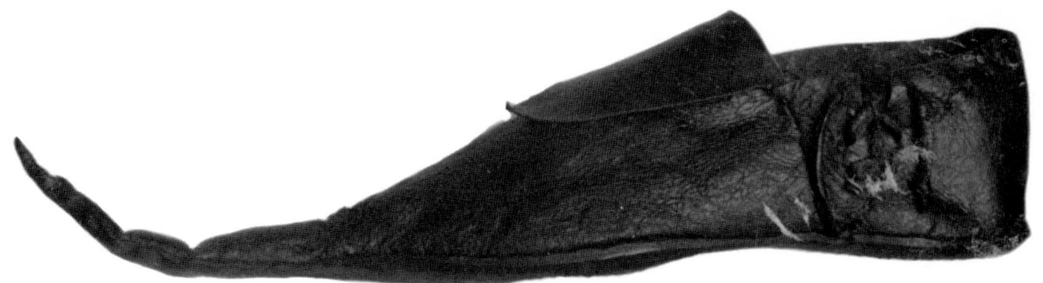

penis sheaths or codpieces. In Europe the codpiece or braquette was first seen in Minoan Crete, later disappearing with the loose Grecian robes and Roman toga. As jackets got shorter in the fourteenth and fifteenth centuries, the pubic region again became visible, and to cover up the shameful area the Church insisted on a modest covering. This modest covering soon developed into the elaborate codpiece, and the exhibitionistic and wealthy introduced the fashion of covering the crotch with a variety of multi-coloured fabrics, padding, bows, jewelry and ornaments. Some kept personal belongings and sweetmeats there. Nowadays, with the jeans cult, a less elaborate codpiece may be seen, particularly among Italians and the homosexual butch.

Like the penis, the foot has been variously deformed, mutilated and decorated. Even today shoes are rarely sold solely as foot covering. Both men and women have always resigned themselves to the discomfort of foot deformation in preference to sensible, sexless shoes. In the thirteenth century, a particular male shoe style called the poulaine developed into the most blatantly pornographic style ever. The shoe had a turned-up toe which gradually became longer and longer, up to twelve inches, and had to be stuffed with moss or cork to keep it erect. It was attached to the knee with a chain to avoid tripping. Some men had the tips designed and coloured as replicas of erect penises, precise in every detail, and used them at more decadent dinner parties for under-the-table titillation. The Church and State both attacked this expression of penile exhibitionism, comparable to the more elaborate penis sheaths of primitive peoples, and the toes were restricted to six inches for commoners and a little longer for nobles!

Only the Chinese lotus foot can compare with the degree of deformation endured by the modern Western foot, which is still compressed into tight, pointed, high-heeled shoes that not only contort the foot but also the torso. There is no rational explanation of why our shoes narrow towards the toes when the natural foot is almost twice as wide across the

above *The foot has been variously deformed and decorated and even today shoes are rarely sold merely as foot coverings. In the middle ages a particular male shoe called the poulaine became associated with the penis. The Church and the State attacked this expression of penile exhibitionism, and toes were restricted to six inches for commoners and a little longer for nobles.*
right *In Europe, the codpiece or braquette was first seen in Minoan Crete, later disappearing with the loose Grecian robes and Roman toga. As jackets got shorter in the fifteenth and sixteenth centuries, and the Church imposed a modest covering, the pubic region became an elaborate display area, often far more self-indulgent than Henry VIII's embroidered codpiece.*

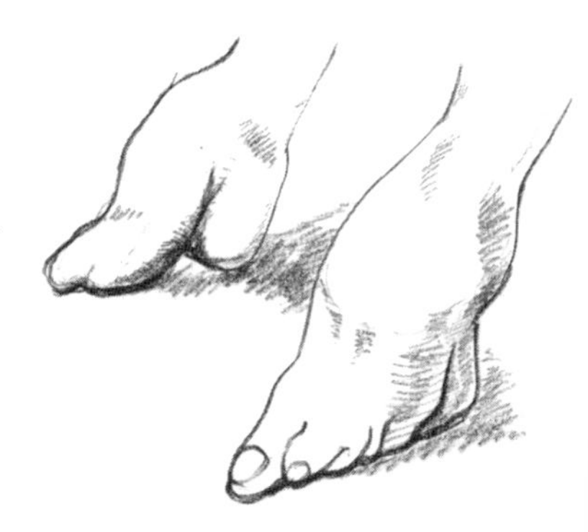

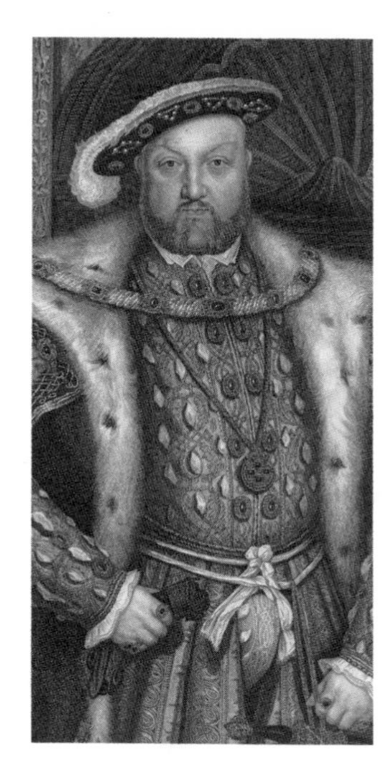

toes as across the heel. When really pointed shoes are in fashion, the *Journal of Podiatry* reports, there is an increase in the business of amputating small toes.

The Chinese bound their women's feet for over a thousand years. They considered them erotic organs to be deformed as other peoples deform the genitalia. This binding process began at the age of five or six, the age when tattooing, scarifying and mutilating women's bodies starts in many other societies. As the girls grew older, the bandages were tightened, and the foot shrank to a fraction of its natural size. The big toe remained unfettered, since it was essential for balance when walking, but the forefoot and the heel were brought as close together as possible, with the four lesser toes curled under the ball. The instep of the lotus foot formed a graceful curve, and created a deep cleft under the arch, which became soft and fleshy. The bound foot represented to the Chinese the very personality of the woman herself. It was obligatory for aristocratic women to have the lotus foot. Unbound feet meant social ostracism and were as serious an obstacle to courtship and marriage as the uncut female genitalia in countries where clitoridectomy is practised.

The lotus foot was used in love-making, and while commoner Chinese women did not necessarily have it, it was considered particularly important for prostitutes and concubines. Even some Chinese men had bound feet: the adopted boys of adult homosexuals, transvestites and female impersonators copied the female lotus foot, squeezing into lotus-like shoes and imitating the sensuous walk. Men found the foot as sexually arousing as Western men find the mouth, the breasts and the neck of a woman. The soft fleshy cleavage under the arch was the equivalent of the labia. It was believed that foot-binding caused a woman's blood to flow upwards, producing voluptuous buttocks and a many-folded vagina. What is more, a woman's feet were the exclusive possession of her husband and even close relatives avoided touching them. To touch was an act of the most intimate nature.

left *Only the Chinese 'lotus foot' can compare with the degree of deformation endured by the modern Western foot, which is still compressed into tight, pointed, high-heeled shoes. The bound foot was obligatory for aristocratic Chinese women and was considered erotic. The binding began at the age of five or six, and as the girl grew the bandages were tightened and the foot was compressed to a fraction of its natural size. The big toe remained unfettered, since it was essential for balance while walking.*

Deforming the waist or the foot is physically harmful. Deforming the head need not be. The skull is a solid case with uniform walls and the capacity of the skull remains the same however alarming the shape into which it is moulded during infancy. All over the world people apply pressure to the baby's soft skull during the first weeks of life to change it according to popular or fashionable taste. Heads are unintentionally deformed by the use of cradle boards or when wrapped in tight swaddling. Intentional methods include the application of special pads, and binding stones and boards to the baby's head.

Head-shaping was practised in pre-neolithic Jericho, in high-born Greek and Roman families, among the Indians in North America, in Africa and in modern Europe. In Egypt, though no deformed skulls have been found, portraits of Egyptian royal families frequently display elongated skulls—consider Nefertiti's bust. At the time of Akhenaten, the royal family and other personages were portrayed in stone and paint with skulls of a remarkable form, and in other parts of Africa skulls have been found of exactly the same consciously distorted shape.

Europe was a great believer in skull deformation. As late as the 1930s, anxious parents in Hitler's Germany massaged their babies' heads to transform the racially despised round head into the favoured long, dolichocephalic, style of the master race. Long heads were already fashionable in the seventeenth century, though for a different reason. A round head would serve as a brain case, but it was held that it did not allow enough room for the memory. 'Let it therefore be longer,' wrote a head-stretcher, 'so that behind it may be elongated like the end of a gourd and then indeed a spacious court is opened where memory can rest.'

In Holland, a rather special head-shape was created by the tight-fitting caps which women wore all their lives and which boys wore until the age of seven or eight. Pressure was constantly exerted on the frontal bone by the longest edge of a triangular headdress and tight ribbons, so that the frontal regions were depressed and inclined backwards. In France, apart from a narrow belt of land north and south of the Loire, the custom of deforming the head seems to have been well-nigh universal up to the eighteenth century. The distortions became so characteristic of certain districts that the forms served as marks of regional identity. French skull deformation was caused by a constricting bandeau worn by babies and children. This resulted in a circular depression commencing from the upper part of the frontal region where it is at its greatest breadth. The forehead was prevented from any upward growth by this bandeau and the skull became flattened, extending behind like the segment of a cone. The newborn child had its head bound in a linen bandage which depressed the skull and also deformed the ear. Children often cried for hours under the application of this constricting

*Ladies in the fifteenth century affected a lozenge-shaped look, not unlike that of the Mangbetu of Central Africa. They achieved this by the shape of the coiffure and by shaving their eyebrows and forehead. ('Portrait of a Lady' by Rogier van der Weyden)*

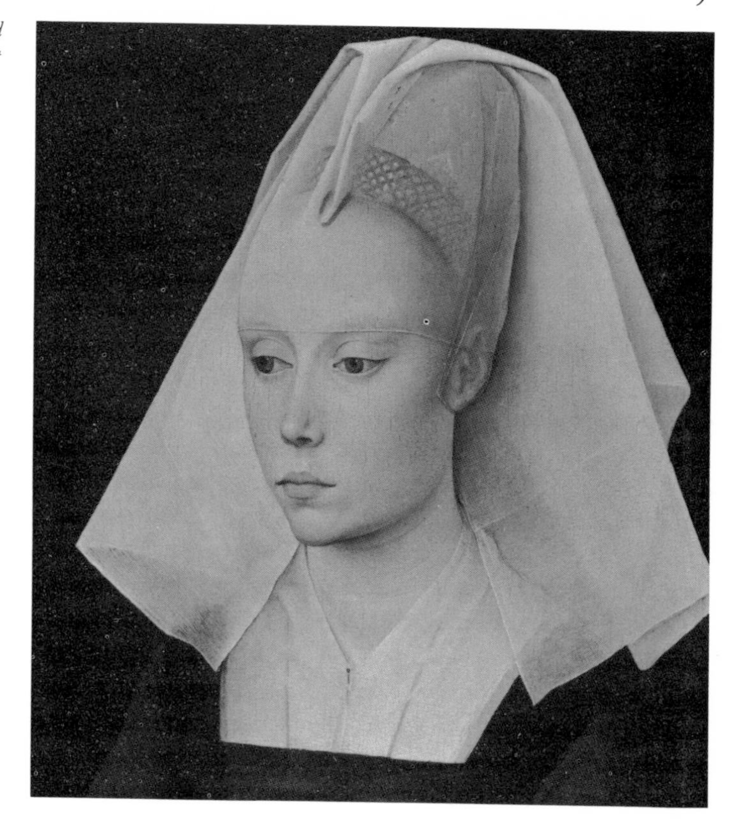

apparatus without the parents realizing the cause of the child's distress. The bandage was seldom removed and harboured thousands of lice which contributed to the development of skin infections and ulcers.

In the Caucasus, as well, heads were deformed by the application of pads and bandages. A little cap lined with wadding was placed on the baby's head closely encircling the frontal, parietal and accipital regions. It was fastened by a band around the head and completely flattened the forehead.

Head deformation, unlike other operations on the body, must be done at birth, and so it cannot be associated with adult passages rites. Outside Europe, cranial distortion is often associated with attempts to separate different groups within a society: castes, classes, slaves. The Brahui Hindus of Baluchistan favour a round head, a broad forehead, a long, thin, pointed nose and small ears. The child's head is wrapped in bandages and kept immobile on a soft cushion; a girl, they say, has holes bored in her ears to prevent her turning over in the cradle and spoiling the work. If the mouth is too large, it is compressed with a small ring; the ears and nose are pinched and pressed. To avoid bow legs, they are strapped together. The trussing of the whole body is done for both aesthetic and supernatural reasons, for should a baby be scared out of its wits by a demon, its limbs would become permanently twisted from fright if they were not tightly tied into the correct position.

The Chinook of the north-west coast of North America had flattened heads. We know from early nineteenth-century drawings that babies were stretched on their backs on a straight plank, attached to one end of which was another flat piece of wood. This fell obliquely over the forehead and was tied down by thongs fastened to either side of the horizontal plank. Another method was to place a board against the back of the head, from the shoulders to a point above the skull. A shorter board was placed on the forehead and the two pieces were tied together with cords, pressing back the forehead and making the head rise at the top, forcing it out above the ears. When these boards were removed at the age of twelve months, the head was perfectly flattened and sometimes the 'peak' of the skull was only an inch in depth. Early observers were disgusted: 'Its little black eyes, forced out by the tightness of the bandages, resembled those of a mouse choked in a trap.' The entire frontal region was flattened and the mass of hair which was forced back exaggerated the idea of a high, back projection.

As the Chinook child grew, the head resumed a more normal shape, though the excessive breadth remained. Among these Indians, slaves were bought from neighbouring peoples. It was only the free-born who deformed their heads; slaves had round, natural, 'ugly' heads, although even they were allowed to elongate their children's skulls. The general shape of the free-born Chinook's head was, therefore, a wedge, with the eyebrows inclined strikingly towards the skull. There was a ridge from ear to ear. And the sharper the angle, the greater the beauty and the more distinguished the individual.

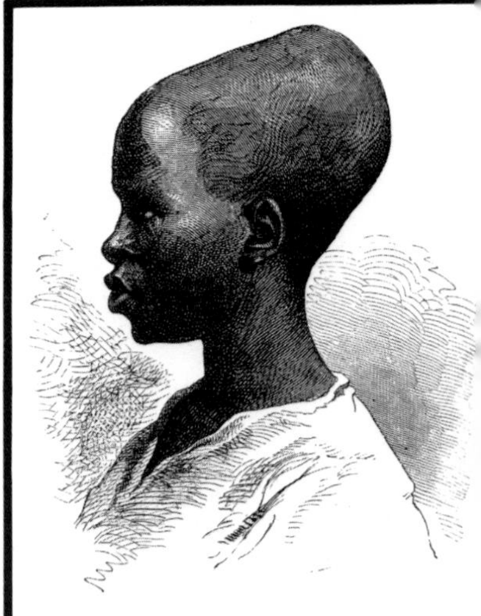

*Head-shaping has been practised since the times of pre-neolithic Jericho. In Egypt, the portraits of royals frequently display elongated skulls. In Central Africa, Mangbetu women had their heads bound to achieve this desirable shape, and a very similar shape can be seen in the skull of a Senegalese youth (from* The Races of Mankind *by Robert Brown, 1873).*

We have seen so far that the body is a clay to be remodelled and a canvas to be decorated. Sometimes the results seem to us grotesque; sometimes beautiful. Usually there is some recognizable motive behind body art which we can at least half recognize. Even in the West the ghosts of primitive instincts still haunt body decoration, but too often they have been exorcised in the name of Fashion and Conformity, and it is on some aspects of these that I want to concentrate next.

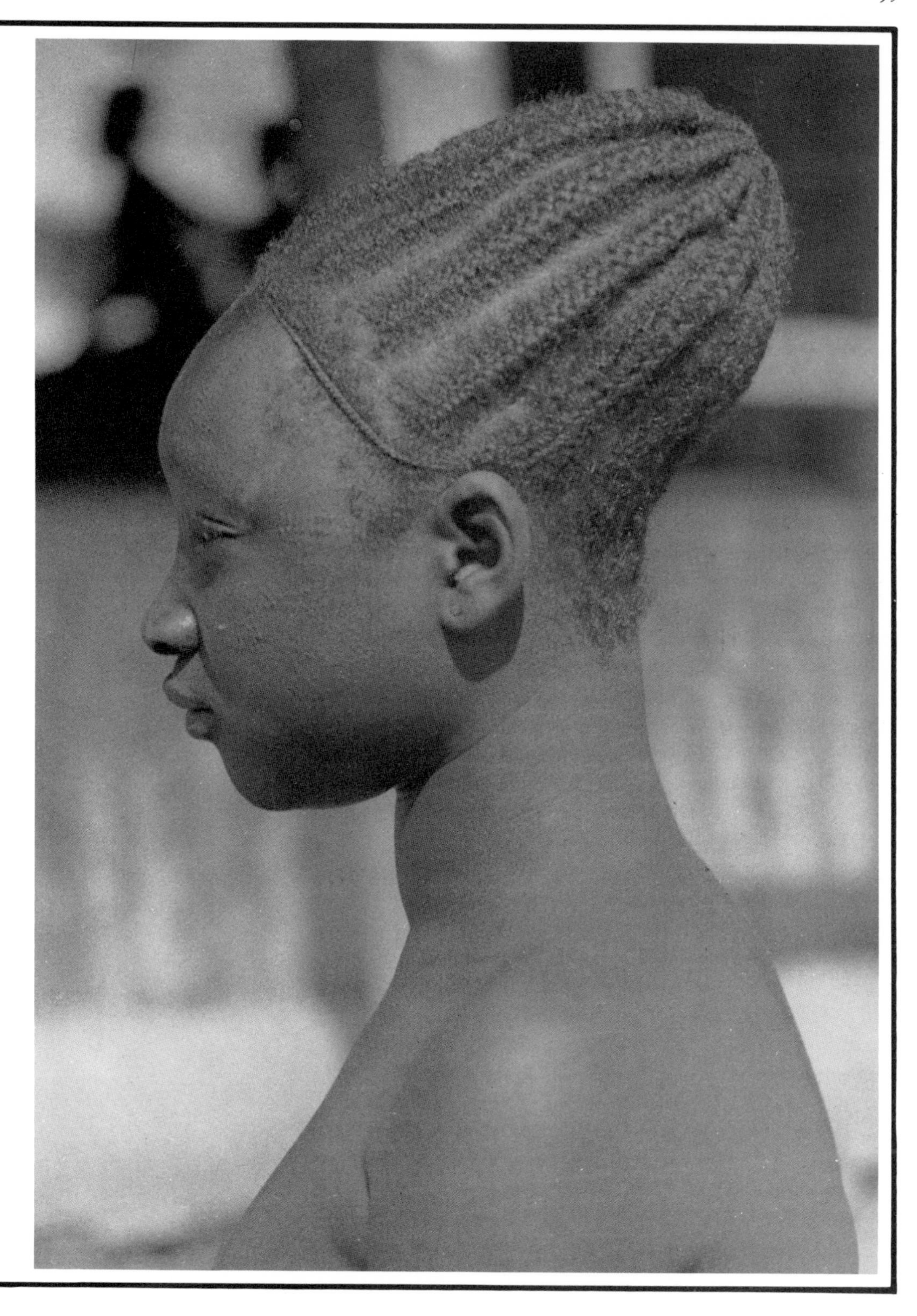

*chapter five*

# The Plastic Body

*Obesity has always been associated with ideas of maternal abundance and erotic desire, and this state was often produced by artificial means—by fattening processes. Fat, particularly on the buttocks, was considered a sign of well-being, as this maternal Andaman Islander demonstrates.*

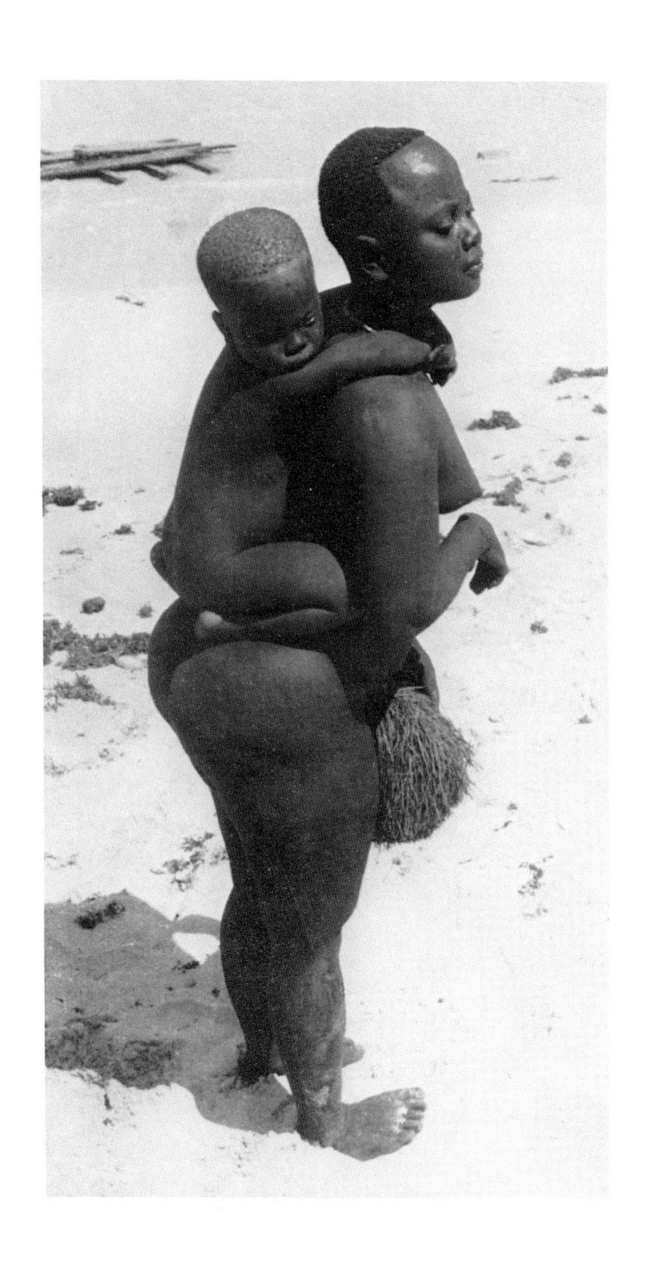

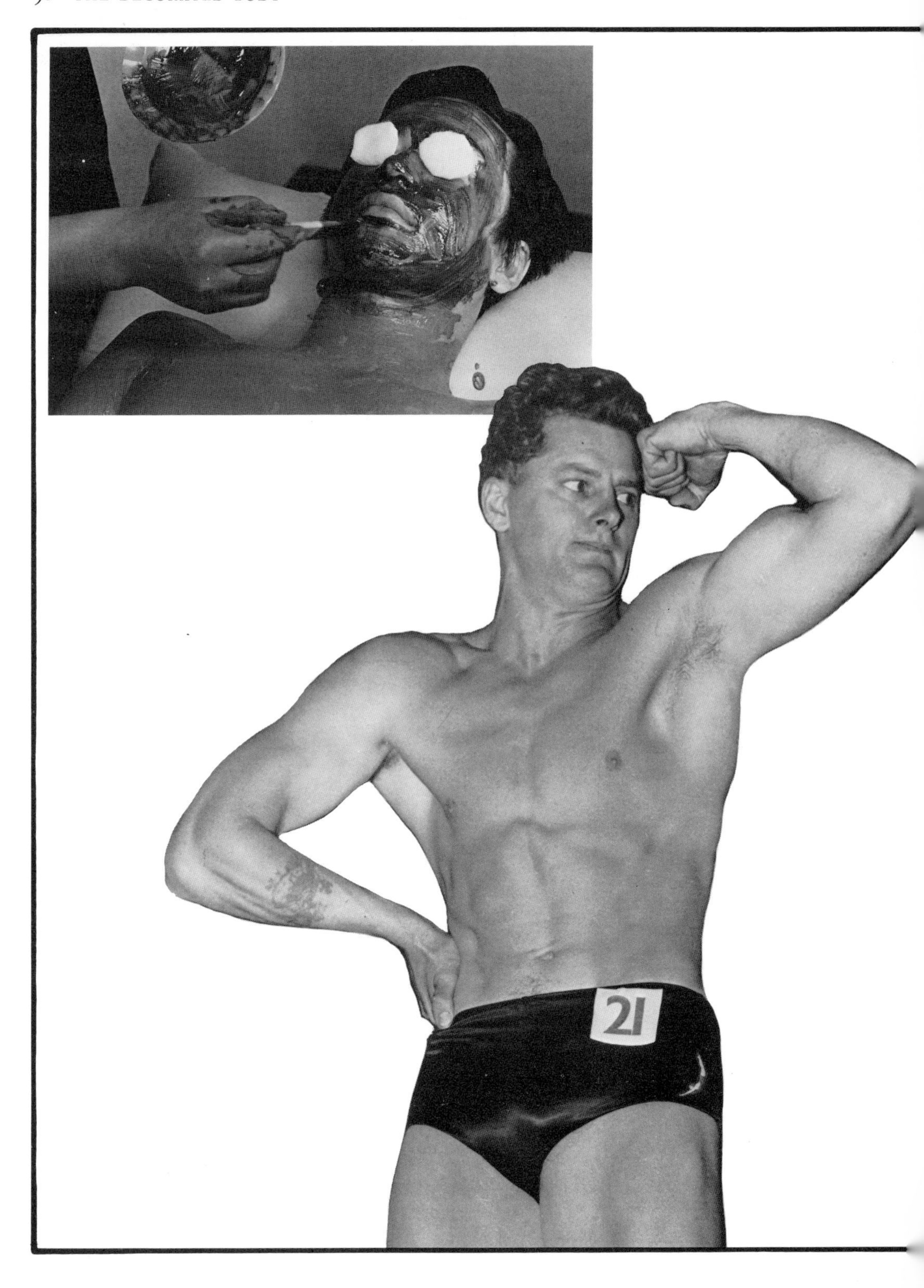
21

top *A facial in a men's beauty parlour in Japan. In most societies men spend as much—if not more—time on beautifying their bodies as the women.* left *Body ideals vary from country to country and generation to generation, men and women learning ardently to become what fashion desires. Body-building is a good manifestation of a Western ideal.*

SOCIETY AND FASHION make their mark on every individual in the West. We learn how to move our bodies to adopt culturally appropriate gestures. We learn a style of walking, a special posture. We wear high-heeled shoes which distort the foot and disrupt the natural balance of the body. We wear corsets which restrict the return of the blood from the legs and may cause varicose veins. We wear jeans so tight that thrush and athlete's foot thrive in the hot environment of the crotch; men are even prepared to undergo temporary sterility as the testicles are pushed up into the body cavity, rendering the spermatozoa infertile.

The Western body ideal may vary from generation to generation, from class to class and from year to year. Men and women learn ardently to desire what fashion desires: fat on the buttocks, fat on the breasts, broad shoulders, drooping shoulders, skin the colour of burnt apricots or of peaches and cream. In some cases the ideal body approximates to the natural. In others it is an entirely unnatural product, outside the grasp of the majority. Whatever the case, as soon as fashion changes, all the pretty girls try to change with it.

In non-Western societies the ideal is not affected by such an ephemeral phenomenon as fashion. The infant is taught to walk properly, eat properly and decorate his body properly, all in a style which that particular society considers 'natural'. The French sociologist Marcel Mauss observed in *Techniques of the Body*: 'In every society, everyone knows and has to know what he has to do [with his body] in all conditions.'

The Fulani in their *gerewol* ceremonies, as described in the chapter on the Sexual Body, promote the ideals of beauty and pride of race. They consider their Negro neighbours inferior, ranking themselves as the 'red' race, the Negroes 'black'. Elsewhere, black may be beautiful.

Similarly, in a Western society which at present favours thinness, a naturally plump body may be drastically reduced by dieting to conform to fashion, whereas in Bangwa (Cameroon) and other parts of Africa fatness is prized in both men and women. Obesity is associated with ideas of royalty and maternal abundance. A plump woman is a desirable woman, and a well-covered girl demonstrates that her family is sufficiently well-off to provide fattening food for her. This plump ideal can in fact only be achieved by upper-class men who have little to do but eat, drink and grow fat, and by nubile girls who are specially 'fattened' prior to marriage. The rest of the Bangwa, men and women, are fit, slim physical speci-

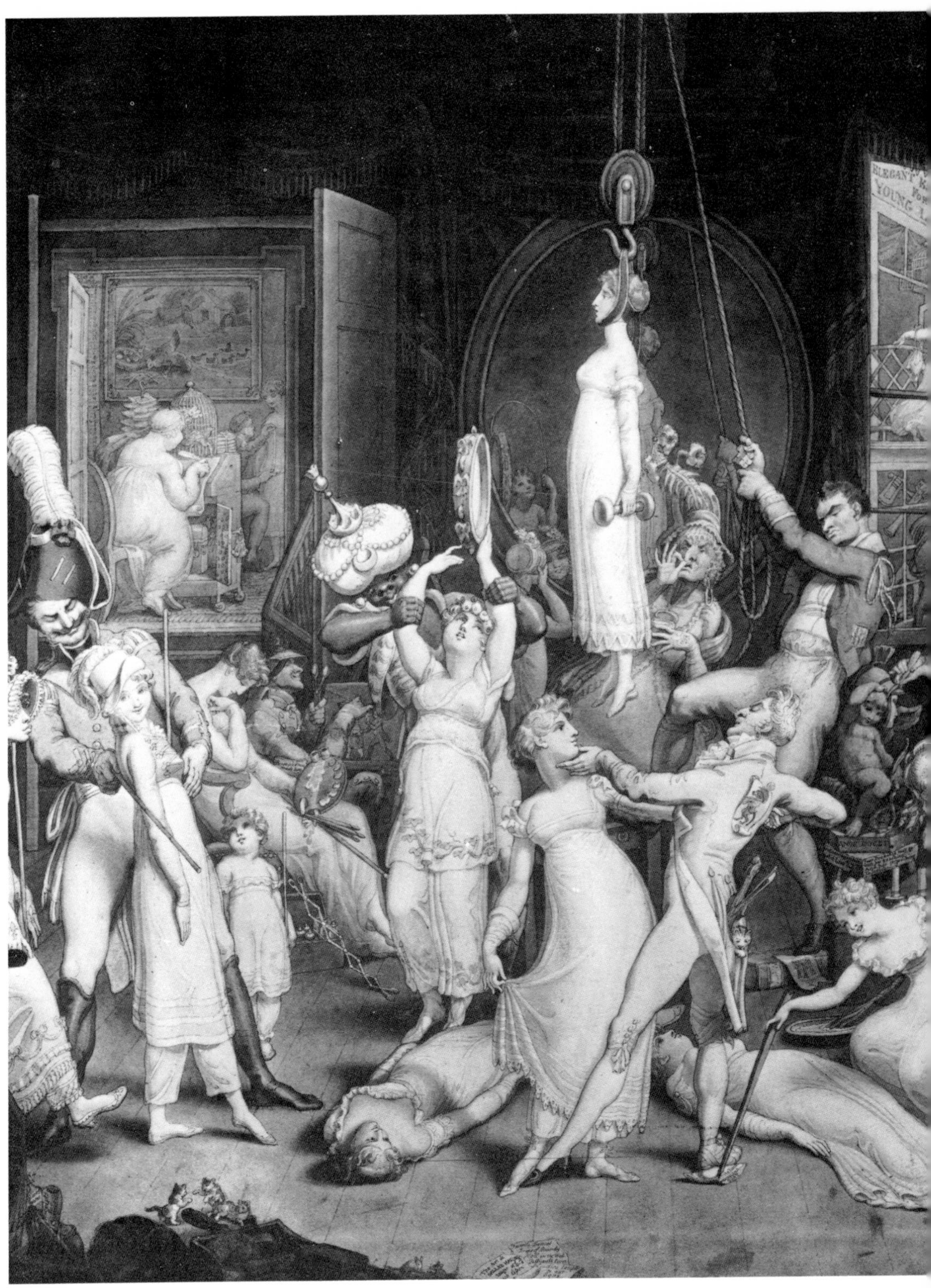

*A beauty school in London*, c. *1800*.

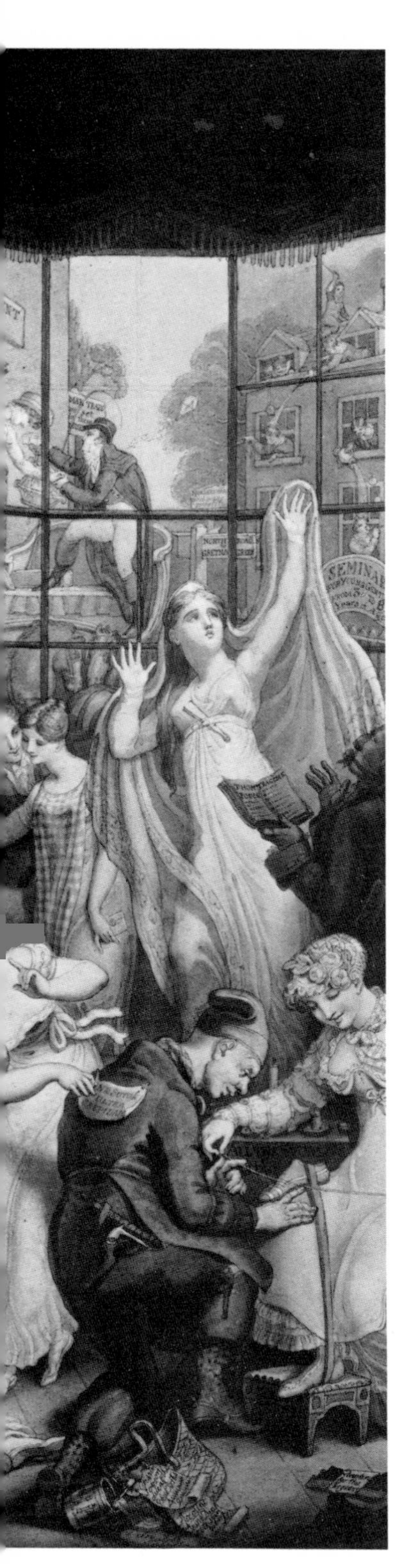

mens, who live high up in the mountains, working in their farms and gardens. In Bangwa, the ideal is fat, the reality thin; in the West, the ideal is thin and the reality often fat. The Bangwa chief, as the focal point of the traditional social system, must try to approximate to the ideal, since his well-being is closely associated with the well-being of the whole community. At the beginning of his reign he is secluded in a ceremonial hut in the palace and 'fattened' for a period of nine weeks. During this time, as well as being fed with the best and most fattening foods, he is anointed with oils and begins to sleep with a few of his wives. During this 'fattening' period the chief is in a taboo state. He speaks only in brief monosyllables and is covered by a blue and white hood. At the end of this period of intense feeding, he takes over his public duties, settling disputes, seeing to the affairs of the country and the elaborately organized palace. At all times he must present a plump, prosperous picture of good health: when the chief is strong and fat, the country is strong and fat.

As far as the women are concerned, their only chance of approximating to the fat ideal is the period before marriage when they spend seven to nine weeks in the seclusion of a 'fattening' house, a kind of cage or apartment where they are fed with delicacies and all kinds of meat and fish until their bodies visibly grow, and their breasts and buttocks swell. The effect is enhanced by a daily rubbing of red palm oil and golden camwood oil. After the period of seclusion and a purification ritual, they are proudly presented by their husbands and kin in the market under a canopy of leaves and a leopard skin. Then they begin to have children and start the arduous life of a married woman, farming and trading. Unlike the Bangwa chiefs their period of fatness is a temporary one.

The contrast with the West is strong. Nubile girls in America and Europe are not expected to be fat-breasted and fat-buttocked as symbols of maternity and pneumatic sexuality. Fatness is a dirty word, a word of abuse, although this has not always been the case. In the nineteenth century, buttocks and breasts were proudly displayed, and middle-aged middle-class men were as proud of their girth as a Bangwa chief, the big belly being a sign of imposing male power. It was a culture trait among German men, for whom fatness reflected wealth and status.

On the whole, however, Westerners have always been a little preoccupied with slimness, devising methods of staying slim while eating as much as they wanted. The Spartans were stern and punitive in their attitude towards fatness. Young people were looked over once a month and those who had gained extra weight were forced to exercise. The Athenians frowned upon fat; Socrates danced every morning to keep slim. Among the Romans the vomitorium permitted men to indulge in excessive eating and drinking, while the women often starved to make themselves thin as reeds.

The West today is an exception to the universal dream of abundance and fertility which has been a human ideal wherever famine is an ever-present possibility and the threat of community extinction a real one. A preoccupation with the quest for food has only been largely eradicated in America, Europe and a few other privileged countries in the twentieth century. Our film stars and fashion models no longer thrill us with their great breasts and buttocks, their heavy arms and thighs. We have learned that fatness, instead of being a sign of good health and beauty, is a sure sign of the opposite. Inspired by advertisements and unnatural ideal types like Twiggy, we set about removing half our bodies in the interest of aesthetics. This passion for slimming rather than fattening has become part of international big business. World-wide organizations such as the Weight Watchers offer special diets and evangelical meetings in order to promote the cult of the thin. Slimming, an American culture trait, is following the Coca-Cola Culture around the world. Even starving India has a Weight Watchers' franchise.

In the 1960s and 1970s, undernourished waifs—fashion models and actresses—have become models for millions of young girls who struggle to achieve an emaciated appearance at the cost of their health, for the thin ideal is an impossible one, at least for the majority of the population. One of the most talked about illnesses of recent times is anorexia nervosa, where young women literally starve themselves in an obsessive struggle to achieve what they imagine is the current body ideal. The anorexic condemns herself to the torture of self-starvation in the futile hope of 'deserving respect' and not being despised for being 'too fat'. The skinny anorexic and the fattened West African are in extreme contrast. The wasting away of the anorexic is a means of refusing to face the anxieties of womanhood in a society where the traditional, even universal, female ideals of sexuality are debased. In West Africa, fattening plumps up breasts and buttocks and brings on menstruation; the anorexic physically prevents herself from developing the normal signs of a mature woman.

*Our film stars and fashion models no longer provide examples of buxom good health. Today half the world is setting about removing half their bodies, inspired by unnatural 'ideal' types like Twiggy, and the passion for slimming has become international big business.*

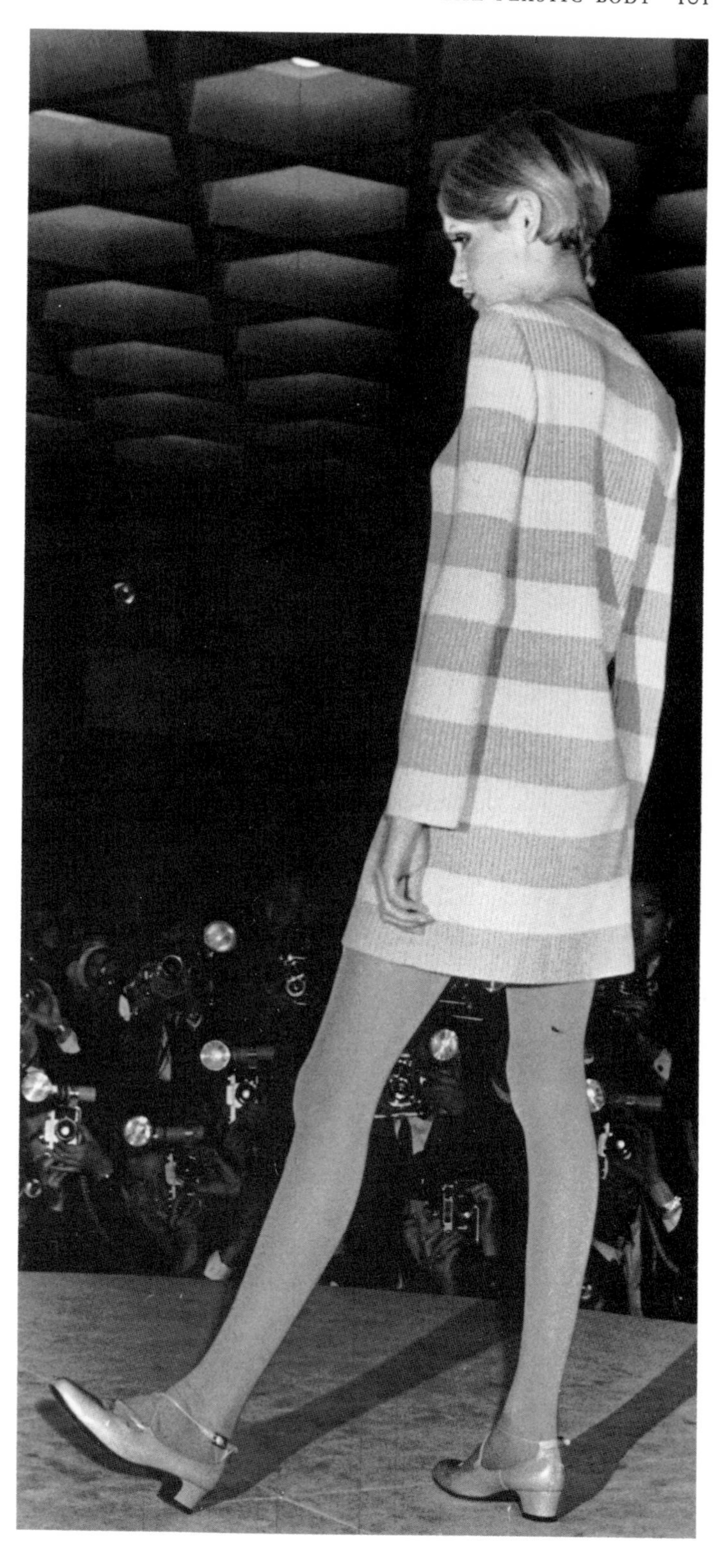

As much as the Fulani, we live in a beauty culture where beauty shops, beauty shows, beauty farms and cosmetic surgery help us to conform to a modern ideal of beauty. If you want success and money and sex and instant approval, you have to join the beauty culture. Nobody will employ you or love you if you are ungroomed, if your age shows in crowsfeet or if your body is too fat or the wrong tint. Millions of very different Americans, seduced by the cosmetics advertisements, look alike, smell alike and walk alike. To be fashionable and beautiful in the global village means avoiding as far as possible any unique character which springs from individual variations such as race, colour or ethnic background. (Most Chinese and Japanese film and pop stars, as a matter of course, have their eyes 'Westernized' by cosmetic surgery.)

Millions of people wear the same skin; young and old are covered with make-up hardened into a theatrical, uniform expression. Millions remove their natural smells and adopt a socially approved mass-produced artificial one. Millions of women have the same shaped breasts. In our excessively visual society disfigurement is crippling: a hare-lip is a cross, the wrong-shaped nose a source of psychological disturbance. Such blemishes are a deviation from the standard, and everything is done to help 'afflicted' individuals to conform as far as possible to the ideal image.

The therapy of human disfigurement advances apace, and some of the most unpleasant operations are performed in the interests of conformity and fashion. Cosmetics become 'pheniatrics'. Cosmetic surgery is considered by health services and health insurance schemes as vital psychotherapy, since it is now accepted that a person's outward appearance can be a handicap to a normal social existence. It has even been decided that criminals who are physically disfigured (ugly!) should have surgical treatment in order to lower the crime rate.

The motives for cosmetic surgery are obviously complex. Some people select a certain part of the body as deformed or ugly as an unconscious method of avoiding their own personality shortcomings. There is no direct relationship between the real degree of abnormality or disfigurement and the magnitude of the 'patient's' need for the operation.

Whatever the reasons, the grotesqueries of primitive body decoration are matched and even outshone by the painful lengths to which we go. In the eighteenth century, the Maréchal de Richelieu 'lifted' his face, since at the age of eighty this libertine still hungered madly after the pleasures

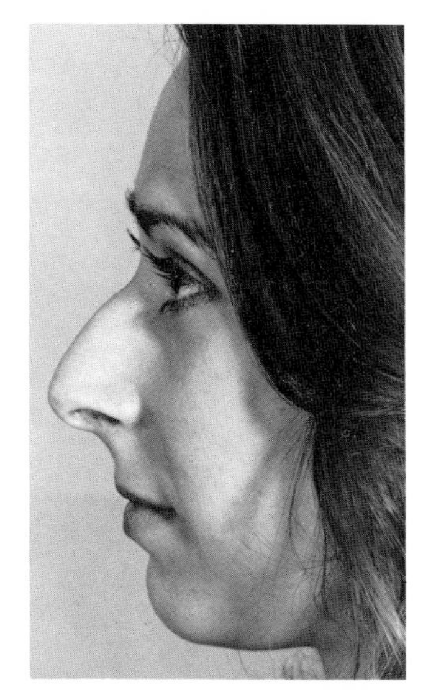

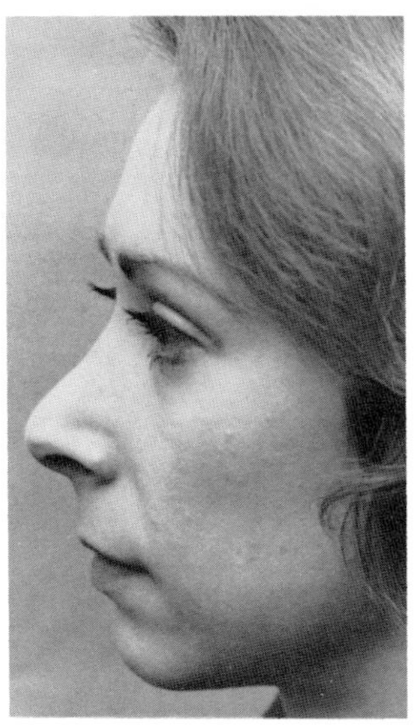

*The nose receives frequent treatment throughout the world, since it is the most obvious of the face's protrusions and is relatively easy to decorate and change. Many societies call attention to the nose. In the West, it is the feature most commonly altered by plastic surgery, usually to make it smaller rather than larger. Changes in identity can be brought about by alterations to the nose, as this case of rhinoplasty shows.*

of love and tried to disguise his decrepitude by a then original method. Every morning he ordered his servant to pull up the skin of his forehead and cheeks and attach the resultant folds firmly to a pad which he wore pinned on the hair of his head. In the sixteenth century, the French surgeon Ambroise Paré made a nose of gold and silver paper and linen cloth glued together. His instructions were that 'it must be bound or staid on with little threads or laces unto the hinder part of the head or the hat'. Paré added: 'Also if there be any portion of the upper lip cut off with the nose, you may also shadow it with annexing some such thing that is wanting unto the nose and cover it with hair on his upper lip so that he may not want anything that may adorn or beautify a face.' He also made eyes of gold and silver 'counterfeited and enamelled to have brightness or "gemmy decency"' which were often held in place by bands of gold and silver encircling the head.

Clearly the sixteenth century was not interested in naturalness. 'Naturalness' today is sought and achieved by brilliant surgery. Overlarge lips can be altered by making a wedge-shaped incision in them and removing the centre. Hare lips can be corrected. Ear lobes are cut down to 'normal' size and jaws made larger or smaller by building up the jaw line or removing excess bone. A modern plastic surgeon can disguise age or rebuild a face to an ideal of beauty. Once performed furtively, plastic surgery is today as acceptable as false teeth, wigs and hair colouring. Moreover, with silicone and similar materials the body is plumped and moulded exactly like clay. Lumps of fatty tissue are removed from the abdomen, the buttocks, the breasts and the sides of the thighs. Hair can be transplanted, using techniques which distribute a significant amount of hair from ageless hair-bearing areas to prematurely bald ones. The whole of the modern Western body can be re-shaped through surgical intervention, the ultimate in body mutilation or cosmetic surgery being, of course, the transformation of an accepted 'male' body into a 'female' one, or vice versa, when surgery and hormones reverse the physical nature of an individual to suit his or her psychological and cultural state.

*chapter six*

# The Symbolic Body

*Modernization means trousers. Few modern states are willing to allow minority groups their idiosyncratic ways of dressing or not dressing. By law, Masai such as these in Tanzania must wear trousers or go to jail.*

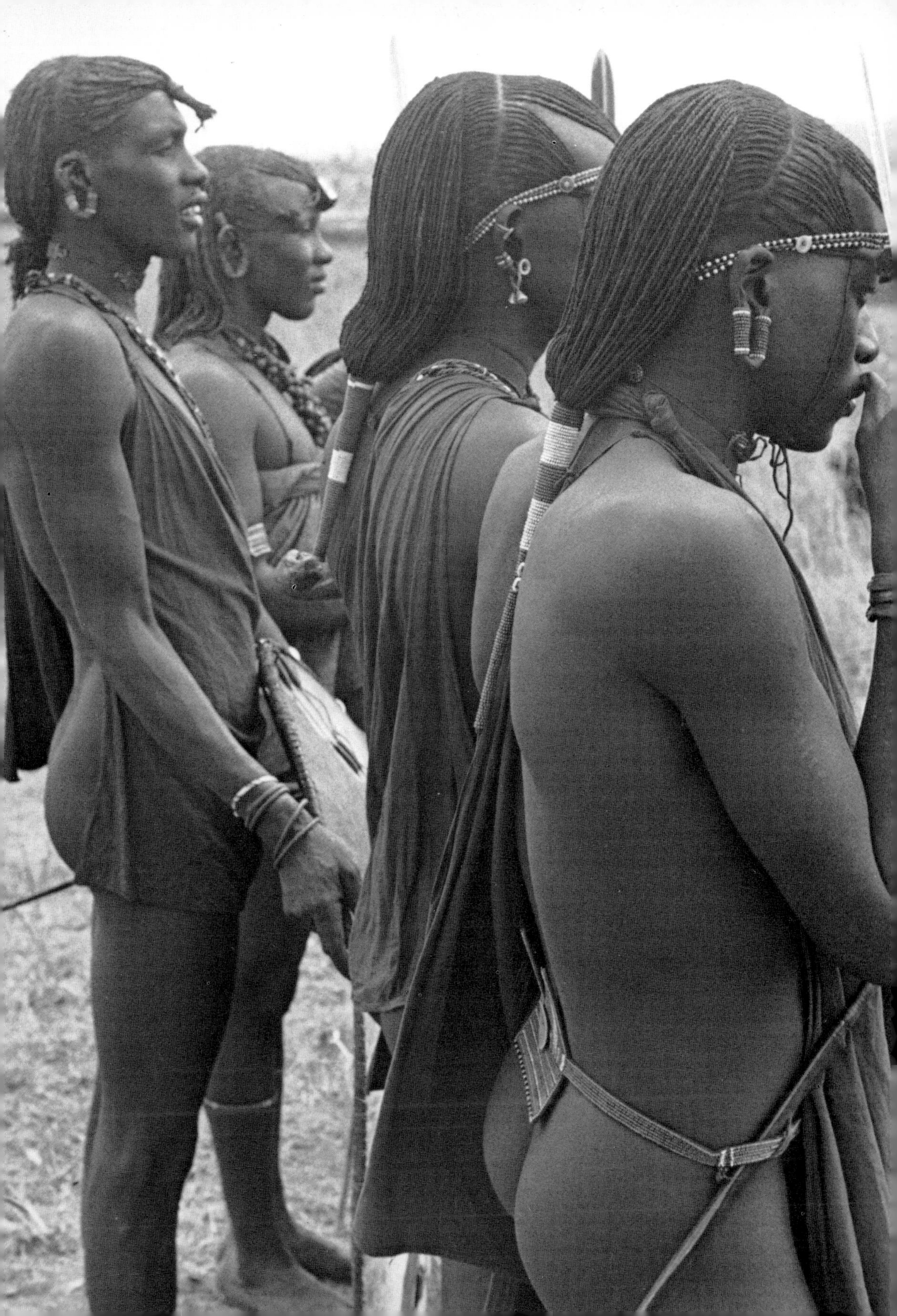

THE CHOICE of body parts to be decorated is never random, but it is only by a study of an individual culture that we can begin to understand such phenomena as the Chinese lotus foot, the 'fattening' of girls, or the prevalent Western interest in the nose and the breast as suitable objects for plastic surgery. In any particular society, features will be stressed at the expense of others. Even erogenous zones dart around the body depending on the culture and chosen not because their nature is intrinsically sexual but because they reflect social ideas.

Travellers have sometimes described in detail the techniques and designs involved in tattooing and scarification, but their social functions and symbolism have rarely been recorded. Even the early anthropologists merely recorded the facts of ornamentation and asked questions about social function. They neglected any deeper meanings, apart from casual suggestions that body art had a magical or supernatural purpose or reflected savage sexuality and vanity.

Sometimes we may discover a direct link with the underlying symbolism. In Northern Cameroon, for example, where lip ornaments are worn by women, the young girls are taught the 'things of women' at adolescence when their lips are pierced. These 'things of women' were first taught in ancient times by the society's ancestress who learned them from a frog. The teaching of the girls gains much from the association of the ancestress-frog relationship with the lip ornaments, since they are said to make the women look like frogs. Among the Dogon, elaborate meanings are attributed to their filed teeth, the twist of leather they wear in their lower lips, the four nostril holes, the pendants of nose beads and the series of earrings. These are all reminders of the mythical origins of weaving and are connected with the actions of their androgynous spirit *nommo*. In other societies eyes may be decorated because they are associated with the soul or 'seeing' in the sense of 'knowing'. Earrings may be linked with the idea of hearing and of behaving well. (The Latin words *obedire* (to obey) and *obedienta* (sounds) are etymologically connected, and the history of the wearing of earrings in the West may be connected with similar ideas.) Yet the Dogon associate the ear with the female sex organs, and other societies protect the ear with earrings as an orifice vulnerable to evil intrusions.

Despite these surface differences, is it possible to discover a universal symbolism of the human body? The body and its various substances play a fundamental part in all symbolic systems, and at first sight there seems to be a similarity in pattern among different societies. A particular symbol, such as the colour red, may have a complex series of meanings, yet there may be a basic one: red may be associated with blood and life. Psychologists have maintained that the meanings associated with basic symbols—such as the colour triad red-black-white—may be related to the workings of the subconscious, which are similar in all human beings. Freudians relate most of them to the sexual impulse. Sociologists prefer to explain universal symbols by referring to the common concerns of all societies: survival, birth, the aging process, the search for food, basic notions of ordering the universe, and sex.

In the study of body decoration, since the practitioners can seldom explain the meaning of the symbols, the explanation has to be advanced by the outsider. But even an anthropologist cannot find out what the symbols stand for in the subconscious of each participant and he has to depend on what they say and relate this to his knowledge of the general cosmological symbolic system.

Most anthropologists, however, would hesitate to accept the existence of a universal symbolism. They would not agree that the foot is universally the symbol of the penis, though it may be so in Western society. In some societies a lot of messy hair hanging down the back may be sexually exciting; in others it may be the sign of a dropout. All human communities have their own map of the body, and they know what the signs are for the beautiful, erotic, magical or socially significant. Body ornaments within a single society are ordered in a complex of signs which amount to a kind of language understood by its members. Among the Bambara of Mali, hairstyles distinguish married from unmarried women, uncircumcised boys from circumcised boys, children of the blacksmiths' caste from the rest. Outside Bambara society, without a knowledge of their body language, the hairstyles could not be read. Even the worldwide practice of circumcision seems to have complex, multiple meaning; there is a vast difference between the circumcision of a Western baby and the circumcision of the son of an African warrior.

One thing which is certain is that within any single society or culture the system of body ornament and the treatment of the body will have an interrelated structure. In the West, the face has always been the focal point of our idea of the personality, probably because it is the only area of the body left totally uncovered by clothing. Eyes, nose, cheeks, ears, chin, mouth neck may be coloured, lengthened, brought into prominence, hidden by make-up, altered by cosmetic surgery, or concealed behind fans, spectacles and veils. In a worldwide context, of all these facial features it is the nose which receives the most attention since it is the most obvious of the face's protrusions and is relatively easy to change. In many tribal cultures the nose is accentuated and adorned. In New Guinea it is ornamented with shells, boars, tusks and feathers. Australians pierced the septum and wore a stick of bone, which helped flatten and widen it, for a flat broad nose was much admired. The Polynesians broke and flattened it. In the West, the nose is the feature most commonly altered by plastic surgery, usually to make it smaller rather than larger. It is considered to be the part of the face which most profoundly affects appearance and personality. Leonardo da Vinci believed that the nose set the whole character of the face, and Dürer showed in his drawings that alterations in its length produced remarkable transformations. Changes of identity can be brought about by quite small alterations to the nose—as has been shown by rhinoplasty performed on war criminals, spies and other people intent on escaping recognition.

We have an obsession about the nose. Other people show greater interest in the neck. In West Africa the neck may be ideally fat or ideally thin, squat on the shoulders or long and swan-like. In parts of Sierra Leone an attractive neck is a fat, plump one that has rings between the collar bone and the chin. Among the Ashanti, women who aim to have beautiful children with long necks carry around with them little dolls, akwa-ba figurines, with long slender necks, which have a beneficial influence on the baby before it is born. Aristocratic women in England had swan necks. The Padaung women of Burma artificially elongated their necks, stretching them by wearing brass rings, the number of which they increased as they grew.

And so on down the body. The navel may be the centre of beauty treatment. Body hair is plucked out. Hands may be exposed to obsessive care, nails clipped close or grown to inordinate lengths. At first glance it would seem that the body is simply decorated where it is most convenient and natural

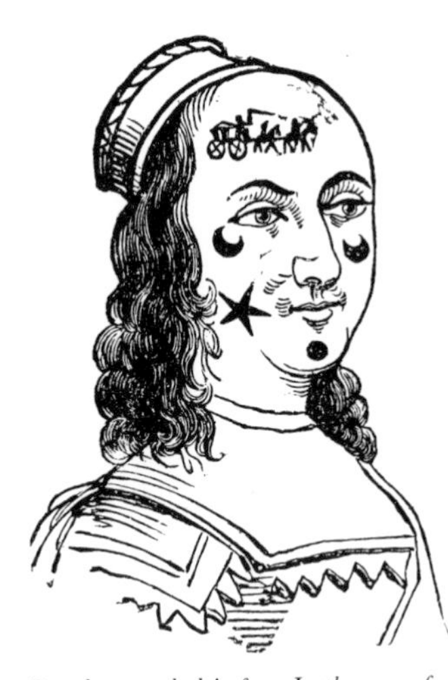

*Patches on a lady's face. In the year of Charles I's execution (1649) a Bill was introduced in Parliament entitled 'The Vice of Painting and Wearing Black Patches and Immodest Dresses of Women'.* right *Lip ornaments add beauty to the mouth as earrings do to the ears. In Northern Cameroon these labrets have symbolic meanings.* far right *Suya tribesman in full war paint with lip plug.*

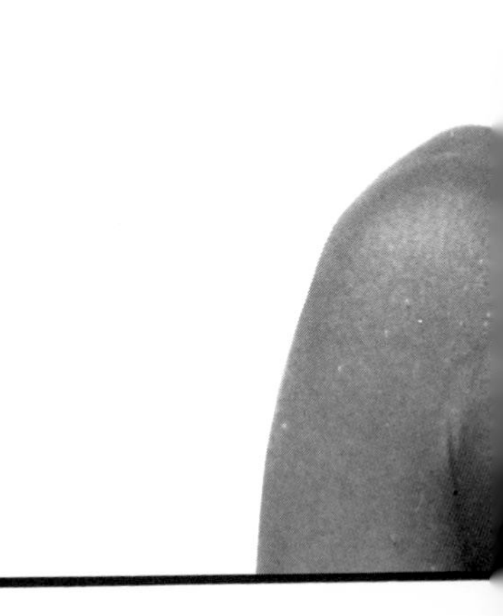

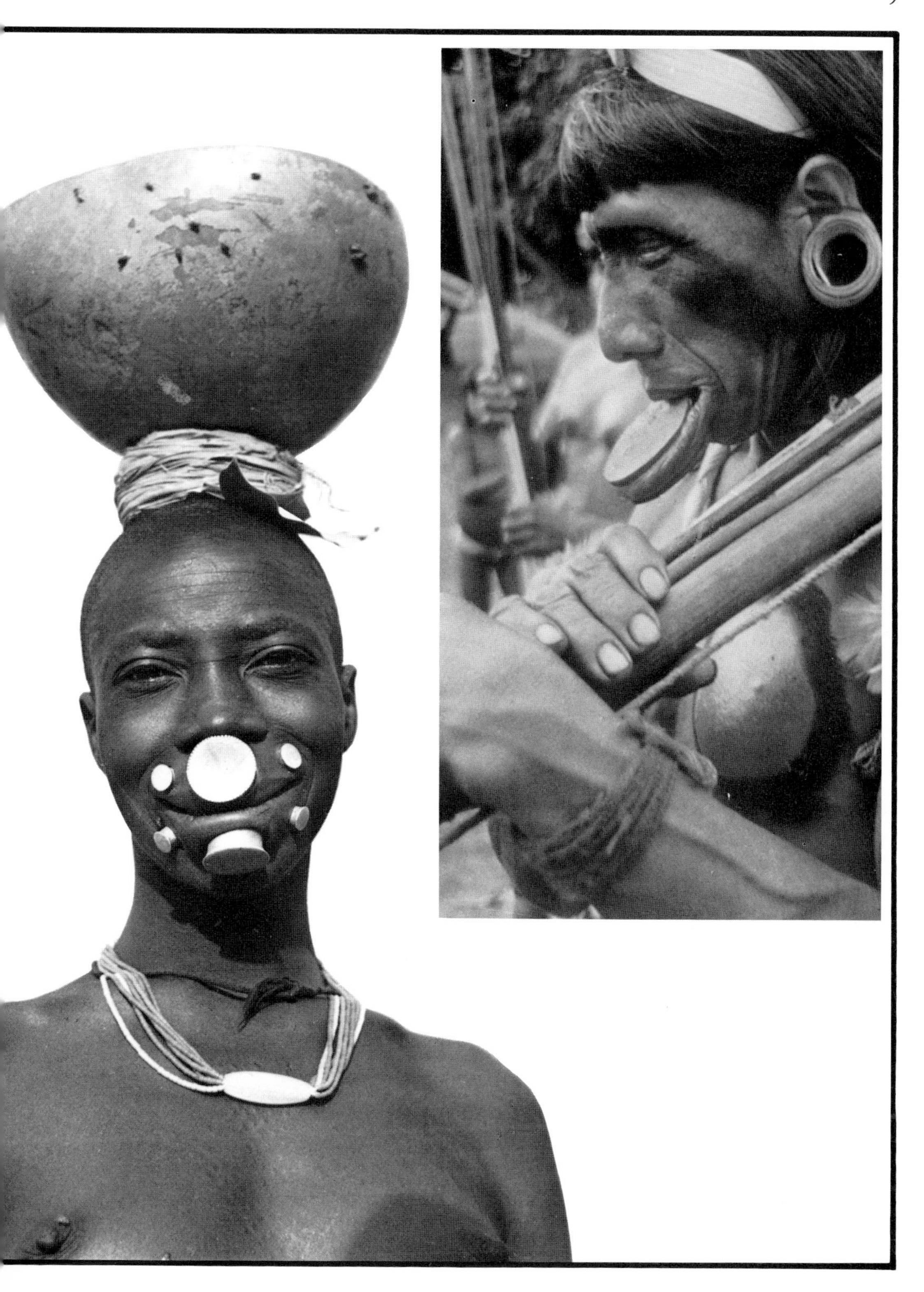

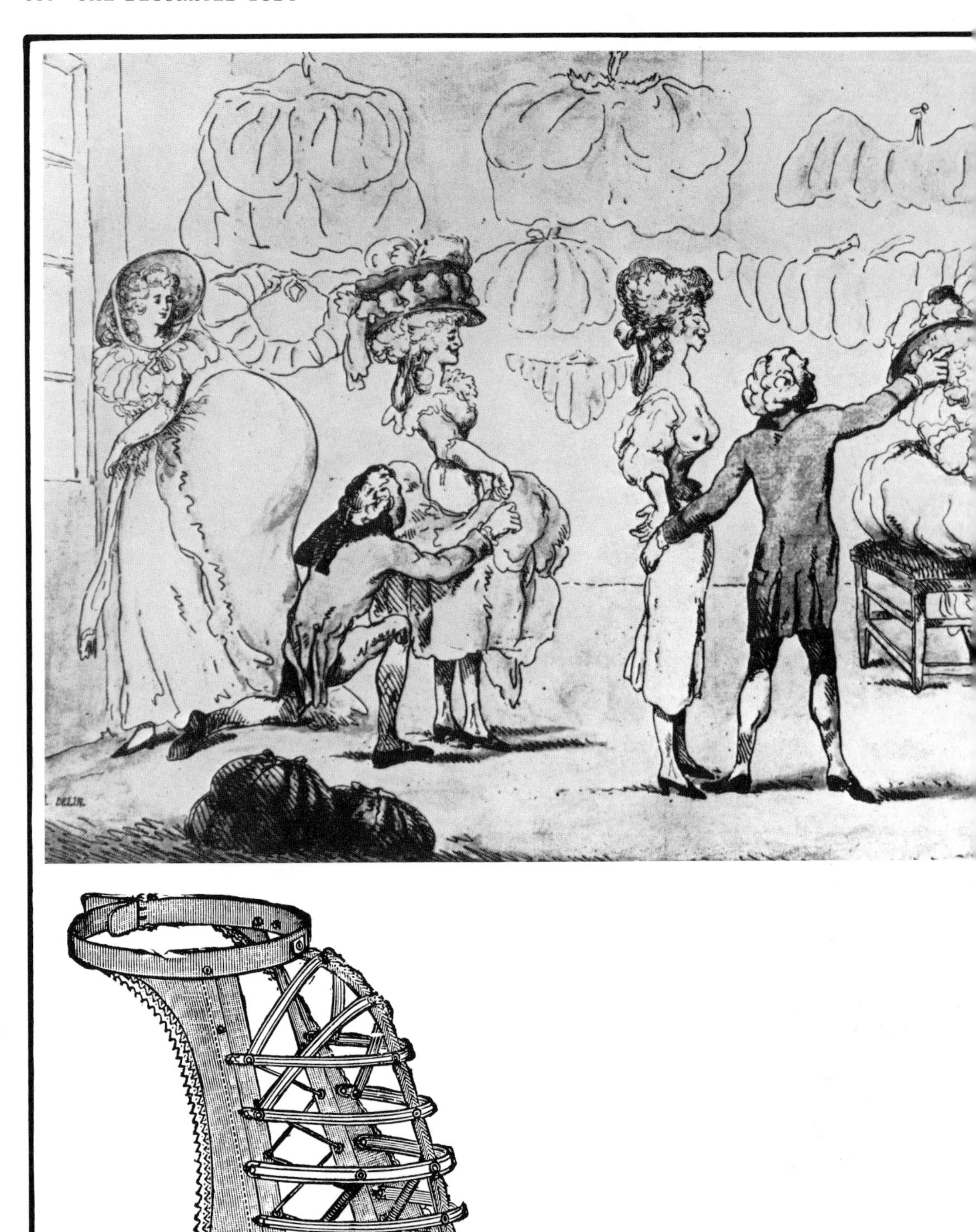

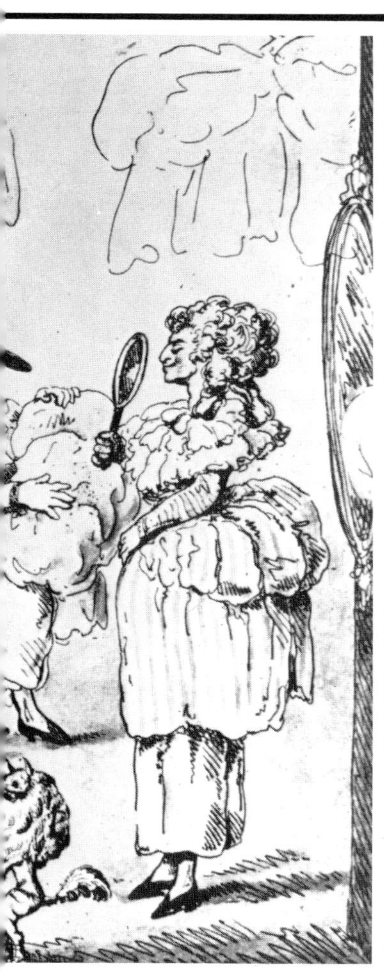

*'The Bum Shop' by Rowlandson. Steatopygia (fatty buttocks) in women has always been admired and the naturally protuberant bottom has been frequently artificially suggested in Western fashions. The bustle* (left) *and high heels have forced Western women to assume an unnatural posture, pushing out the buttocks and accentuating their motion in walk.*

to decorate it, or where the parts are most attractive. However, these areas are no more 'natural' or aesthetically pleasing than the pierced noses, restricted calves or excised vaginas of exotic peoples.

The Western attitude to the breast is a case in point. Once upon a time, breasts were a symbol of maturity and maternity. The oldest representations of the female form date back to the Paleolithic period 30,000 to 20,000 BC, and are statues of obese women with large breasts and abdomens, such as the Venus of Willendorf found on the shores of the Danube. Other figures present steatopygia (large buttocks) as an aesthetic condition. In sculptures of the Neolithic period, and in those of the prehistoric Greeks, Babylonians and Egyptians, there is an obvious admiration for women with large breasts and buttocks. In many societies, buttocks are the symbol of fertile womanhood. The Bushmen and Hottentots of southern Africa admired a characteristic steatopygia in their women—fatty buttocks caused partly by the backward curvature of the spine at the sacrum, which make the pelvis rise almost vertically. This natural protuberant bottom has been suggested artificially in European fashions by the bustle, and by high heels which force women to assume, unnaturally, the Bushman posture, pushing out the buttocks and accentuating their motion in walk.

Until recently, the mature, maternal body was extolled in the West in painting and sculpture. Even today large bosoms may be admired, though not because they represent fertility or maternity but as a measure of sexual potency. Prudery and fashion prevent a woman displaying her buttocks or her private parts, so she makes her breasts a prominent sexual characteristic that cannot be overlooked. The female breast has long been a focal point of erotic and aesthetic treatment. In Egypt, courtiers bared their chests in summer, painting their nipples and outlining their breast veins in blue. Prior to the 1920s, the bold bosom was emphasized by tight corseting in Europe, and even artificial shadows and pale blue paint accentuated the cleavage of Edwardian women.

To us it is part of the order of things for a woman to accentuate her breasts or at least present them in a fashionable, 'sexy' way. A stranger to our society would be at a loss to explain the symbolic significance of a firm, round bosom on a woman of sixty, particularly if milk glands were not, for him, erogenous zones.

The problem of understanding body decoration in its

cultural context has been taken up by some anthropologists. Anthony Seeger, while not attempting to compare the symbolism of body ornament in 'civilized' and 'primitive' societies, has looked at closely related South American communities, which vary in their elaboration of body ornament and the parts of the body which are decorated. His purpose has been to try to understand the interrelationship between symbolism and ornament and the body. Among the Gê-speaking peoples of the Mato Grosso in Brazil, he found a lot of attention paid to the ears, the lips and the eyes (and the penis), and this ornamentation seems to have reference to ideas about hearing, speaking, seeing and sex. Lip, earlobe, nose and penis ornaments are worn throughout the area, but some tribes wear ear-discs and no penis sheaths; some pierce a hole in a man's lower lip; others prefer to hang feather ornaments in the ears.

Seeger has been able to show that the decoration of a certain organ is related to the symbolic meaning of that organ in the various subcultures of the Gê groups. The ornamentation of the ear, rather than the mouth, indicates the symbolic importance of that organ in one society. The ornamentation of the mouth may stress the importance of 'speaking' in one society rather than 'hearing'. These ideas may easily be applied to Western associations with the body parts, such as the breast or the mouth.

Among the Suya, a Gê sub-culture, ear-discs are worn in the ears of both men and women, supported by thin loops of distended ear-lobes. They are large discs of wood or palm-leaf spirals. Men often don't wear their ear-discs during the day, wrapping their lobes up around the ear itself, rather as a housewife leaves her hair in curlers or under a scarf when she is in the house for the day, fluffing it out for public and social occasions. However, the Suya man never goes long without his lip-discs, removing them only to wash—perhaps in the same way as many married women in our society never take off their wedding rings. On ritual occasions the Suya wear new lip and ear ornaments, adorned with tassels, strings and other elaborate appendages.

It would appear that in Suya society it is the faculty of speech which is being emphasized, as opposed to the faculties of sight and vision. The eye is not important or at least not as important as it is in Western society, where it is elaborately decorated and thought of sometimes as a 'window of the soul'. The Suya see the eye as the locus of the dangerous and antisocial, and dreaded forces associated with witchcraft are thought to enter the body through the eyes. Similarly, the Suya give very little attention to the nose, at least to the nose opening. The sense of smell is associated with animals rather than human beings, and the nose is left severely alone as far as decoration is concerned.

Thus the Suya stress the ear in their body symbolism, and the ear-discs are supposed to help people to hear and 'understand things', to 'know things'. For men, rather than women, the lip-disc has important symbolic associations with aggression and warlike attitudes, which are again linked with masculine self-assertion in oratory and singing. In the case of the lip and ear ornaments, the colour rather than the form seems important: red is specifically associated with heat and belligerence and is used for lip-discs, while white, associated with coolness and passivity, represents the idea of listening and knowing and is the colour of the ear-discs. The third 'universal' colour is black, which the Suya associate with witches and antisocial attributes, and it is used as paint on the eyes and nose, specially during hunts and ceremonies.

Face ornaments, ear-discs and lip-discs are also linked with different phases in the growing-up of a Suya youth. Ears are first pierced at adolescence, while the lips are pierced only when the adolescents become fully adult. Becoming adult is associated with ideas about hearing and speaking, and the acquisition of these important 'social' faculties is thought to be fully achieved with the wearing of discs. Children with unpierced ears are not expected to 'know' or 'understand' anything, just as they are not expected to behave in an adult way. At puberty, however, when their ears are pierced, they are expected to listen seriously to their elders and follow their instructions. The bigger boys have their lips pierced when they enter the men's house and leave the world of women; and while they are waiting to marry they learn songs and continue to insert bigger lip-discs.

Through the wearing of ear- and lip-discs, the body is socialized and the ornaments are closely related to fundamental ideas about the social personality, morality and the symbolism of body parts. Neighbouring people, related to the Suya, emphasize different social artifacts and different parts of the body, since their notions of morality and concepts of the person differ fundamentally from the Suya. The Shanate, a Central Gê group, receive penis sheaths at puberty, and social control of young men is symbolized by this demonstration of the control of a youth's sexuality. Instead of stressing ear- and lip-discs, knowledge and the spoken word, the Shanate seem to use the penis sheath to indicate sexual potency and at the same time the social control to which dangerous sexual powers are submitted.

The Suya case makes it clear that in some societies at least it can be demonstrated that the use of certain ornaments and certain colours are closely related to a culture's symbolic and social system. But it does not make any contribution to the theory of a universal symbolism. Can one, for instance, associate the colour black with evil and death, and red with blood and life, and white with the spirit, cross-culturally? Some observers have pointed out that colour symbolism is culturally relative and usually have given the example of the colours used by Westerners and the Chinese in mourning. But the question of why we wear black and the Chinese wear white would seem to be irrelevant, and I suspect that the wearing of white in China can be explained by a more detailed analysis of Chinese funerals and colour symbolism, white possibly symbolizing hope, or the ancestors or spirit. In ritual, black is almost universally associated with death, evil, dirt and danger.

The basic colour triad is found in all body decoration and is available to all peoples. Black is readily at hand to those who have fire, red is obtained primarily from iron oxide, and white from clays and chalk. Among the Thompson Indians, whom we have already examined, red symbolized the good life, heat and earth; black, the opposite of red, signalled evil, death, bad luck and darkness; white represented the world of the spirit, ghosts, dead people (as opposed to death). For the Tchikrin of South America, the three colours had specific roles; red was linked with health, energy and sensitivity; black with transition, danger, and death; white meant purity, transcendence over the normal world.

Red seems to have a special significance everywhere. Apart from the fact that it is the colour of blood and is readily procurable, red is the primary colour with the longest wavelength perceptible to the human eye, the colour with the greatest natural stimulus value. In Australia, red ochre was the most important colour in their widespread cosmetic industry and the most popular source was the ochres made by exposing iron oxide to the heat of fires. Deposits sometimes served large areas, and when one community did not possess its own natural resources, supplies were obtained from neighbours, even enemies. Some groups made expeditions of hundreds of miles to get the red ochre.

In Tasmania, the women were the miners, levering out the iron ore by gripping a stone in their hand and using it to strike a sharp-pointed stick into the rock. The ochre was packed in wallaby skins and distributed by trade and barter around the island.

On the Australian mainland, ochre was carried from tribe to tribe in oblong parcels of bark. Small quantities were always carried by the men, either in their chignons or in their dilly bags. Ochre also had a magical significance on the mainland. When a group arrived at a mine, the young men, under the guidance of an elder, removed all their ornaments, cut their beards and threw the hair towards the pit, running to hack the ochre and then running away with it without looking back. Ochre—the bloodstone—is explicitly associated with blood by the Australians, and the two substances are closely related in myth. Ochre pits are supposed to be the blood-stained scenes of the death of ancestral heroes. Blood itself is used in rituals and body ornament. The men make a small longitudinal cut through the skin and puncture the vein beneath it lengthwise. The blood spurts forth immediately and is collected in the handle-pit of a shield. Blood is applied to the body with a small brush, and usually acts as an adhesive.

In other parts of the world, red may be obtained from trees and plants. Among the Bangwa, the precious red camwood powder is obtained from the bark of *Sacocephalus diderrichii*. In the African savannah lands and in areas influenced by Islam henna is used. Henna, like antimony, has the triple merit of being medicinally helpful, having a beautiful colour, and being religiously desirable. Said to be Mahomet's flower (the Egyptian privet *Lawsonia inermis*), it is used as a cosmetic and as a means of purification or protection from evil influences as well as a medicine.

René Caillie wrote in *Travels through Central Africa to Timbuktoo:*

> This henna . . . is found in great plenty in the interior: the Moorish women bruise the leaves and obtain from them a pale red tincture which they use to brighten their charms. The leaves being bruised and reduced to a pulp, this pulp is applied to various parts of the body which they are desirous of staining; it is kept covered, to preserve it from the action of the air, and moistened at intervals with water in

> which camel dung has been steeped. The colour is five or six hours in fixing: after that time the pulp is removed and the flesh to which it has been applied is stained a beautiful red. Henna is applied to the nails, the feet, and the hands; upon which last they make all sorts of patterns; I have never seen it applied to the face. The colour remains a month without changing, and does not disappear entirely in less than twelve months. It is not only an ornament with the Moors, but a religious ceremony for women who are about to be married. When a woman has used henna she takes care to show it, and to attract attention to her hands and feet, that she may be complimented: women are coquettes all the world over!

An anthropologist, Victor Turner, has suggested a profound significance for the universal preference for the colours red, black and white. He suggests that among the earliest symbols produced by man are these three colours, which are symbolic representations of the products of the body. These colour-products are in turn symbolic of important social relations. White is linked with semen or mother's milk and hence reproduction. Red is associated with blood and hence with the mother-child tie, or war and hunting. Black is seen as excreta or decay and associated with death or a transition from one status to another, which may be envisaged as a temporary mystical death.

In this way the colours are made to stand for basic human experiences of the body and provide a classification and symbolism of these experiences involving reproduction (red—blood), suckling (white—milk) and defecation (black—excreta). This colour triad is of universal significance:

> The three colours white-red-black . . . are not merely differences in the visual perception of parts of the spectrum; they are abridgements or condensations of whole realms of psychobiological experience involving the reason and all the sense and concerned with primary group relationships.

Equally interesting as a symbol is hair. Hair makes an admirable social and sexual symbol. It is clearly visible; it is easily manipulated; it is not painful to cut; it grows, so that transformations are only semi-permanent; and it can be shaped into forms of sexual and social adornment. You can

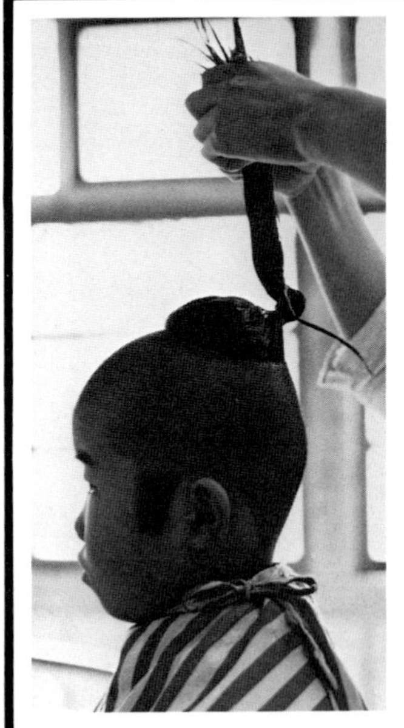

*The top knot is a classic Japanese hairstyle which has completely fallen out of fashion.* right *In Africa, hairstyles indicate a woman's status as unmarried girl, married woman, mother, mother of twins, widow. Hairstyles, as in the West, however, may simply be a matter of fashion, as in the case of these three Iko girls.*

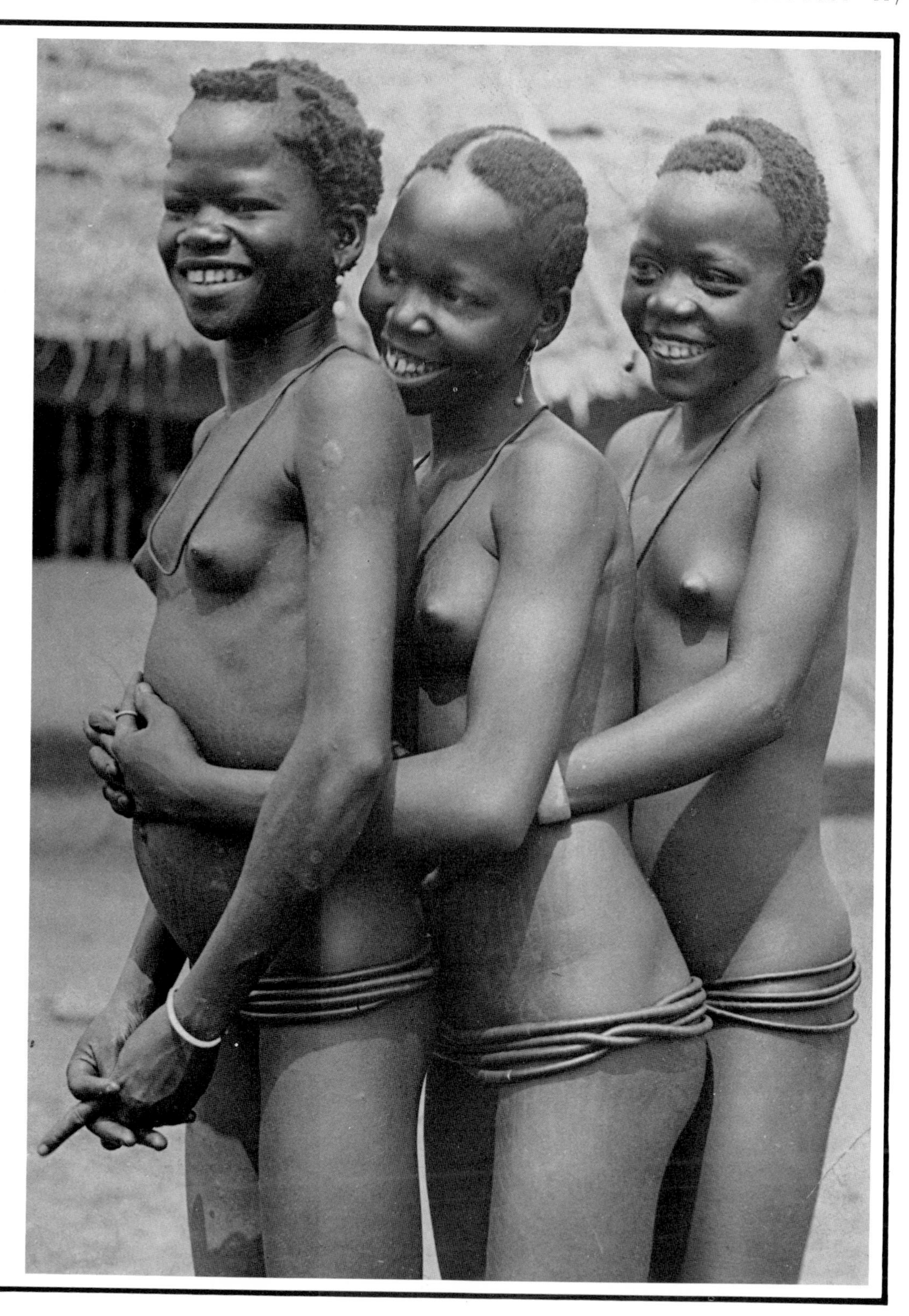

do many thousand things with hair: pleat it, plait it, frizzle it, topknot it, construct it into monuments, remove it, tonsure it, dye it or straighten it. The Egyptians wound it on wooden sticks, covered it with mud, and baked it. The Masai built up their hair with clay and thread; Bangwa women shaved it off; the Ibo shaved their heads, allowed the hair to grow to a uniform length of a quarter of an inch and then cut it into geometric patterns like figured velvet.

Hairstyles can represent social groups. Among the Bangwa, if a woman had long hair she was a mother of twins; slaves had traditional hairstyles; so did royals. Hairstyles may indicate relative age: Omaha boys had their heads shaved close with tufts; men either wore their full head of hair or shaved if off except for a continuous roach along the sagittal line. In our own society, the tonsure signified a ritual state and nuns cut off their hair. Hairstyles distinguished men from women, and in the West until recently the symbolism was so strong during this century that long-haired men were considered effeminate and short-haired women mannish. It used to be the custom in our society for young girls to wear their hair down and post-adolescent girls to wear it up. In this way hairstyles still tell us a lot about people: good boys and nice girls have neat hair, crewcuts and bobs, while bad boys and naughty girls have long loose hair.

Hair is a mysterious substance. Long hair may be associated with strength as in the case of Samson, with wild force as in the case of Esau, with sexuality, or with asceticism and spiritual power as in the case of the prophets. The state and treatment of hair definitely indicates a kind of social condition. In the West, short, cropped hair signifies acceptance of discipline: convicts, soldiers, priests and others 'under orders' have short hair. The compulsory haircuts forced on the long-haired defendants in an English obscenity trial (the *Oz* case) seem a clear example of the disciplinary message conveyed by hair. Totalitarian governments are always nervous of long hair, and it may be forcibly cut by the police. In 1967 the military dictators of Greece announced that long-haired tourists were no longer welcome, and Julius Caesar in subduing the Gauls made them cut their hair as a token of submission.

Hair is used in ritual and magic since it is seen as an extension of the whole person. A man in mourning may shave his head to remove the impurities of death as well as to demonstrate a sense of loss. The Greeks cut off their hair and

right *Hairstyles and beards were regulated by sumptuary laws in Ancient Egypt. (Cairo Museum, relief on limestone sarcophagus,* c. *2000 BC).* below *American woman in the streets of Philadelphia. A fashion in high, lacquered hair requires an exotic preparation.* below right *Hairstyles can tell us a good deal about people and about the societies they live in. This engraving, 'Fashions in hair', was made in 1788, the year before the French Revolution.*

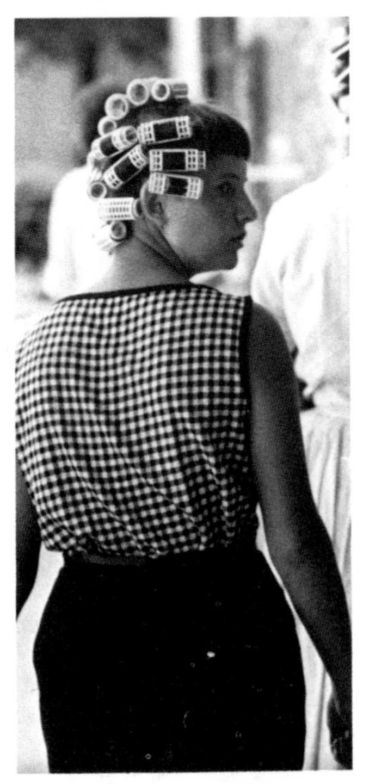

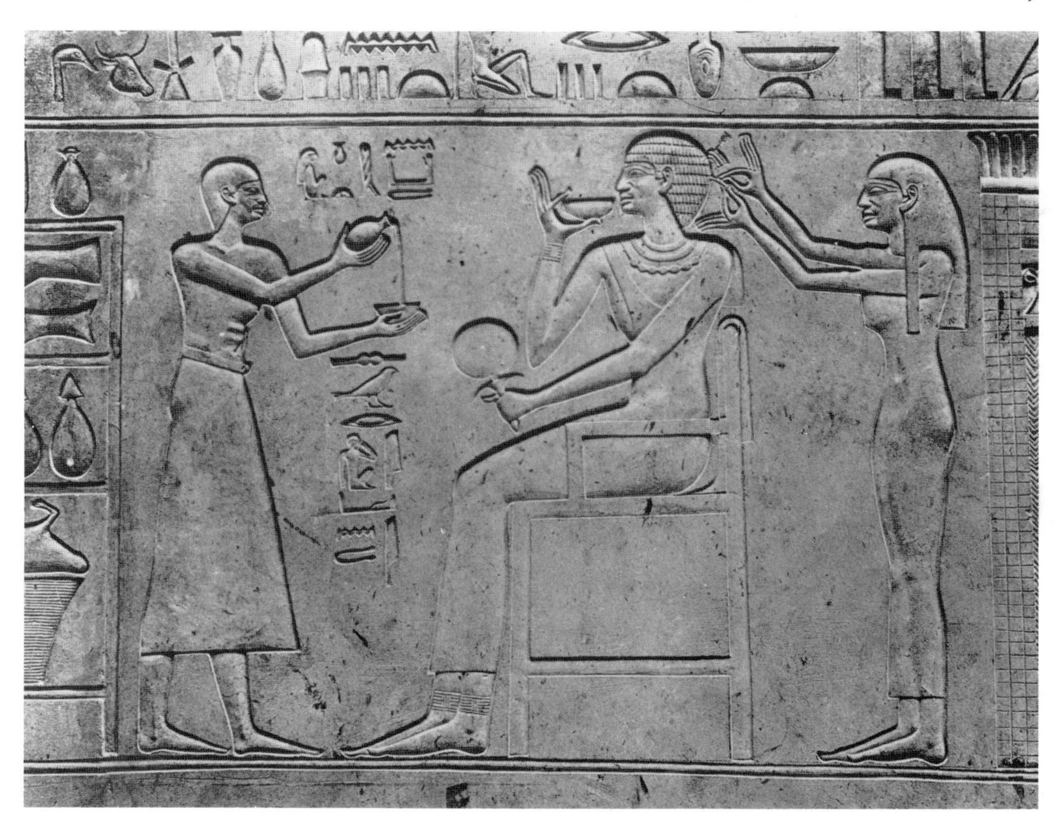

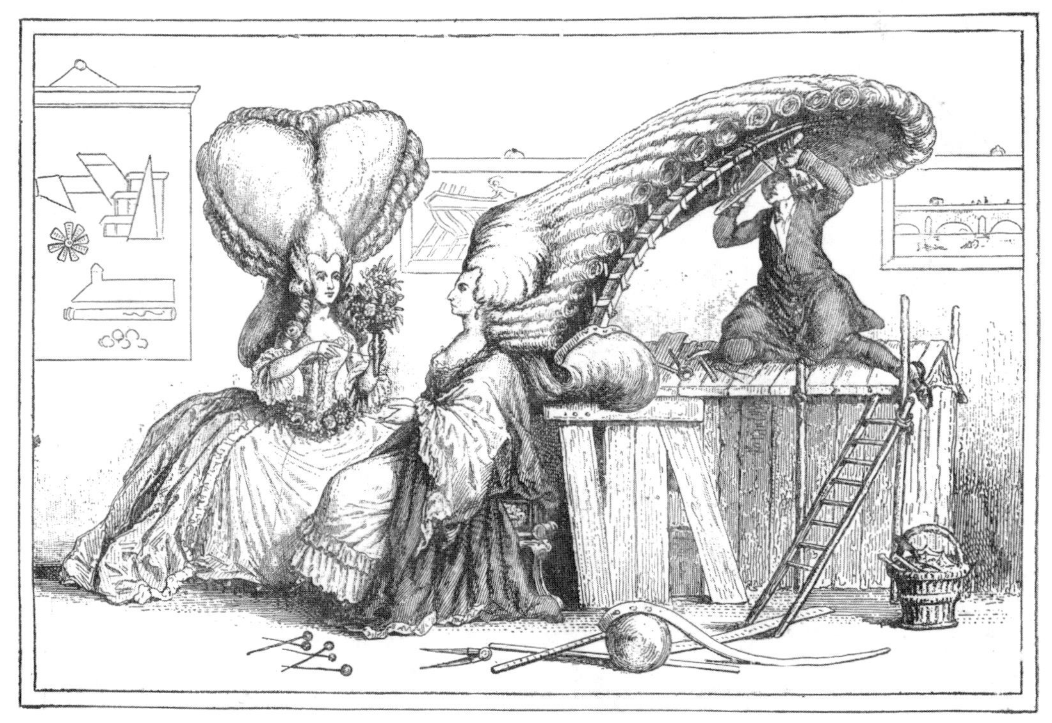

laid it on the corpse. The Hindu ascetic keeps his head shaven to symbolize his total rejection of all bodily and worldly pollution. However, in Hindu society, as well as the shaven-headed ascetic, there is another type of holy man who leaves his uncombed, uncut hair in a long matted mess as a manifestation of the sacred. In fact all high-caste Hindus go through a period in their lives when their hair is left matted: from birth a Hindu boy's hair is never cut until the day of the tonsure, when it is cut and given as an offering at the shrine of a god. So there are two basically opposed ways of achieving a state of sacredness, either by shaving the head and rejecting the world (as in the case of most monastic orders) or, like the prophets, leaving the hair uncut and becoming subject to ecstasy and divine possession.

Hair may be a symbol of sexuality and pollution or the very stuff of sacredness. The Greeks saw the head as the source of male semen in the form of the cerebrospinal fluid and considered the state of the hair as an indication of a man's sexual vigour. The psychologist Charles Berg, followed by some anthropologists, considers hair as a universal symbol of the genital organs, a bodily symbol which gains its strength through this association with the genitals. Hair is seen as phallic—either as the actual penis itself or as the semen. As a result, if hair is used in ritual the meaning is usually phallic.

According to Berg, then, hair is a phallus, the only one that convention permits us to wear in public. (In a way it corresponds to another stretched idea: that the painted mouth is the woman's vagina.) Untidy, upstanding hair is socially unacceptable, since it represents the penis, and a respectable, socially acceptable gentleman should comb his hair neat and flat.

A woman's hair is more easily recognized not as her genitals but as a substance imbued with sexuality. In church, long tresses were once covered. In the Middle Ages, the anti-sexual attitudes of the church were seen in their disapproval of long hair; women's hair was considered provocative and tied up in wimples. If a Hebrew woman untied her hair and uncovered it she was considered shameless, and even today some orthodox Jewish women crop their hair at marriage and afterwards conceal their natural hair from the sight of everyone except their husbands; once they wore the shetel but nowadays it is likely to be a perfectly ordinary wig. A woman's sex belonged to her husband and so did her hair.

One of the most valuable possessions of the Australians

was the hair of their wives. Most of it was spun into string, but it was used for special purposes also such as making shoes. An Australian had absolute rights over his wife's hair and could cut it whenever he chose.

Hair, like bodily secretions such as sweat, blood, and urine, is a magical substance in the thought of all the peoples of the world, since these substances which leave the body are thought to remain in contact with it when abandoned and retain a mystical association with it. Since hair grows constantly (even, according to popular belief, after death), it is associated with life and vitality and its use in sacrifice is convenient, since cutting it off causes no pain and sheds no blood.

The symbolism of body art is not a subject on which one can be dogmatic. It is easy to theorize about it; difficult to be factual. The 'symbolism' is so often associated not with deep, sub-conscious meanings but with more simple effects, such as animal mimicry or sexual arousal.

*chapter seven*

# The Sexual Body

*Western cosmetics, imprisoned by the phenomenon of fashion, do not celebrate in symbol the physical and social body. They celebrate sexuality, vanity and the conformity to fashion's dictates.*

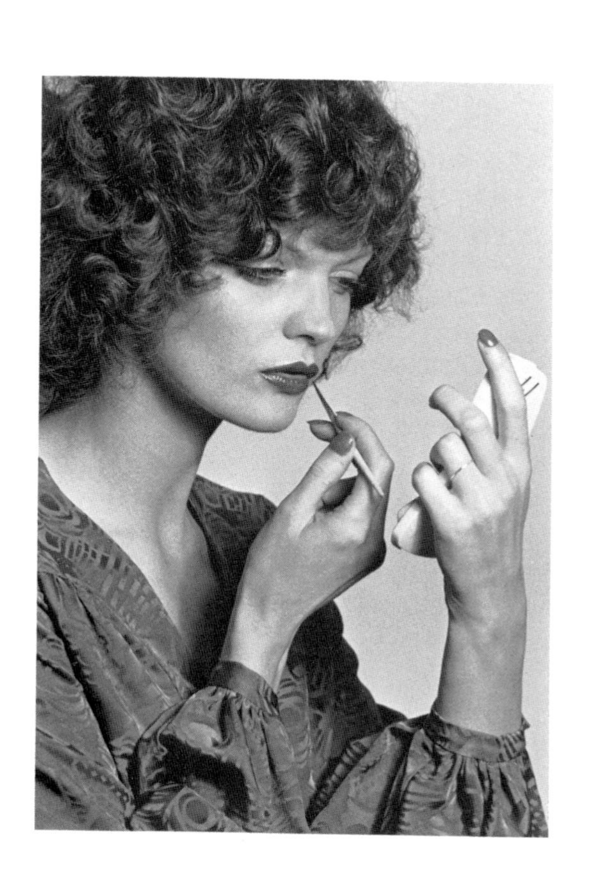

PAINT AND TATTOOS protect both the primitive and the civilized from the unknown. Until recently, interpretations of body art were distorted by Western attitudes to cosmetics and to the primitive. Primitive society was magic-ridden, therefore painting, tattooing and scarification must have a supernatural origin. On the other hand, Western society was rational, therefore the only explanation a Westerner could give for the need to decorate the body, particularly the face, was a sexual one.

Painting in the West has always been associated with lust and immorality. Body decoration, paint, clothes and tattoos may serve to embellish the body, presenting it reshaped and rejuventated—a young, attractive image for all the world to see.

Human beings, unlike other animals, are constantly on the arousal. In the West, sexual messages are coded and sent by an elaborate combination of clothing, ornament and body decoration. Non-Western people also employ decoration to transform the neutral body into a sexually attractive human body. To those who practise tattooing, an untattoed body is naked and an unsuitable object for physical passion.

Body decoration may sometimes seem blatantly sexual, even though this is not the whole story. When well-meaning missionaries from Europe provided the Tasmanians with clothes, it was in the belief that they would happily leave off their 'mess' of ochre, charcoal and grease. But they misunderstood the point of the decoration. The Tasmanians fought against wearing clothes. Their women, they said, refused to have sexual intercourse with them if they did not wear their paint.

In the West, cosmetic displays are no longer restricted to special occasions. Society does not insist that its members show themselves painted only on ordained festivities, times when erotic impulses ordinarily kept under control, can be released.

On the other hand, it was on special occasions that the Caduveo women painted their bodies with erotic spirals and whorls, using abstract motifs to present the body in an oddly asymmetrical but exciting way.

This 'decorative dislocation', according to Levi-Strauss, combined aesthetics with a subtle element of sexual sadism which may explain the appeal of the Caduveo women, who attracted many European outlaws and adventurers to the shores of the Paraguay River. Several of these men, then very old, described to the French anthropologist, with great emotion, the nude bodies of these adolescent girls completely covered with interlacings and arabesques of a 'perverse seductiveness'.

Obviously body decoration is frequently blatantly sexual. Many scarification and tattooing marks draw attention to erogenous zones: breasts, buttocks, thighs. Much body decoration converges on the genitals. But there are forms of erotic body decoration which are not so appealing to the Westerner. Maori women, for instance, made themselves attractive by tattooing their lips and chin; they said that 'naked' faces appeared shrivelled, old and ugly. Polynesian women stain their lips and darken their teeth in order to attract men; to them, European women with white, unfiled teeth and pink lips are ugly, like dogs.

In Africa, both men and women stress the excitement of a beautifully scarified body—the special sensitivity of the scars on a woman's belly or thigh. These marks embellish the body, reshaping and rejuvenating it, in order to present an attractive, sexually satisfying image. Decoration can also disguise or hide unattractive features, thus helping to achieve a degree of consonance with society's idea of the 'beautiful' and 'sexy'.

North-west of Alice Springs in Australia, Walbiri women paint each other's bodies for sexual as well as ritual reasons. Discussing the significance of the paintings, they stress that the designs are aimed at men, and that they make their bodies appear fatter and their breasts larger. While these designs often have a deeper significance, the women stress sexuality and vanity: they paint and dance to attract a lover. Like the Western woman, however, the Walbiri woman paints not only for sex: she paints for her own general satisfaction; she decorates when she goes food gathering with her friends; she paints as a celebration of her *general* female sexuality.

Australian men, too, paint to attract lovers. Cosmetic paintings among the Australians are quite different from the ritual paintings at initiation rites and increase ceremonies. Their compulsion is exercised in physical terms. The designs on the body and the songs sung are thought literally to draw a woman towards her hopeful suitor. (Western cosmetics promise similar results for those who wear certain scents or lipsticks.) Hearing the chanting in her sleep, a Walbiri woman is supposed to find her stomach made 'sick with desire'. She will get up and follow the song and the painting. These paintings are mainly practised in youth; when asked why older men gave up this type of decoration, they explained that it would be shameful, even silly, for old people to call attention to their undesirable, aging bodies.

Apart from painting himself, an Australian will also paint his wife, to keep her faithful and prevent her defection to another man while he sleeps. The same designs are painted on a new wife or when a man leaves the camp for a journey, worried about his wife's fidelity.

*Husbands and wives in the Andaman Islands decorate each other's body. Their motivation is symbolic protection as well as vanity and sexuality.*

Sexuality can be a major ingredient of a certain kind of body art. In the *Kama Sutra* we are told that women should be skilled in the sixty-four cosmetic arts, including the colouring of teeth, nails and bodies, and tattooing. In South America, the Toba, a group related to the Caduveo, always painted when they were in the mood for love. Along the Rio Guapes, the Desana paint their faces with barred lines interspersed with crosses and circles, interpreting the circles as drops of semen, symbolic of friendship. The men decorate themselves to ensure luck in hunting, which they express as 'making love to animals'. The face is painted with figures of prey and the signs which represent semen, and the animal is seduced into being killed. Likewise a shaman puts an imaginary design of red paint on his patient's body in order to attract the sexual attentions of the healing spirit.

Tattooing, in Japan, had a subtle but frankly erotic effect, particularly in the case of the celebrated courtesans of the past. Even today a Japanese prostitute may have herself tattooed with a snake coiling about her groin about to take refuge. Her breast may be tattooed with full-blown peonies, the inside of her thighs decorated a delicate pink.

Japanese men tattoo their genitals. The penis becomes a peach, a plum or an eggplant, the full detail of the design only becoming visible when the penis is erect. During tattooing, the men maintain tumescence for long periods. Other erotic designs are tattooed in white on the body so that they only show when the skin is pink after a hot bath or when flushed with excitement. The Japanese associate tattooing with sexual arousal. In one eighteenth-century novel, a Japanese woman speaks of the delight of making love with lower-class men with their patterned bodies. An old poem written by a woman of rank speaks of her delight in the body of her lover, comparing herself to a bird hovering over a wonderful landscape of blossom and strange beasts. There is no doubt that even in the industrialized West making love to a tattooed body may

*The achievements of the West in body painting are tawdry compared to the aesthetic success of many primitive peoples.*

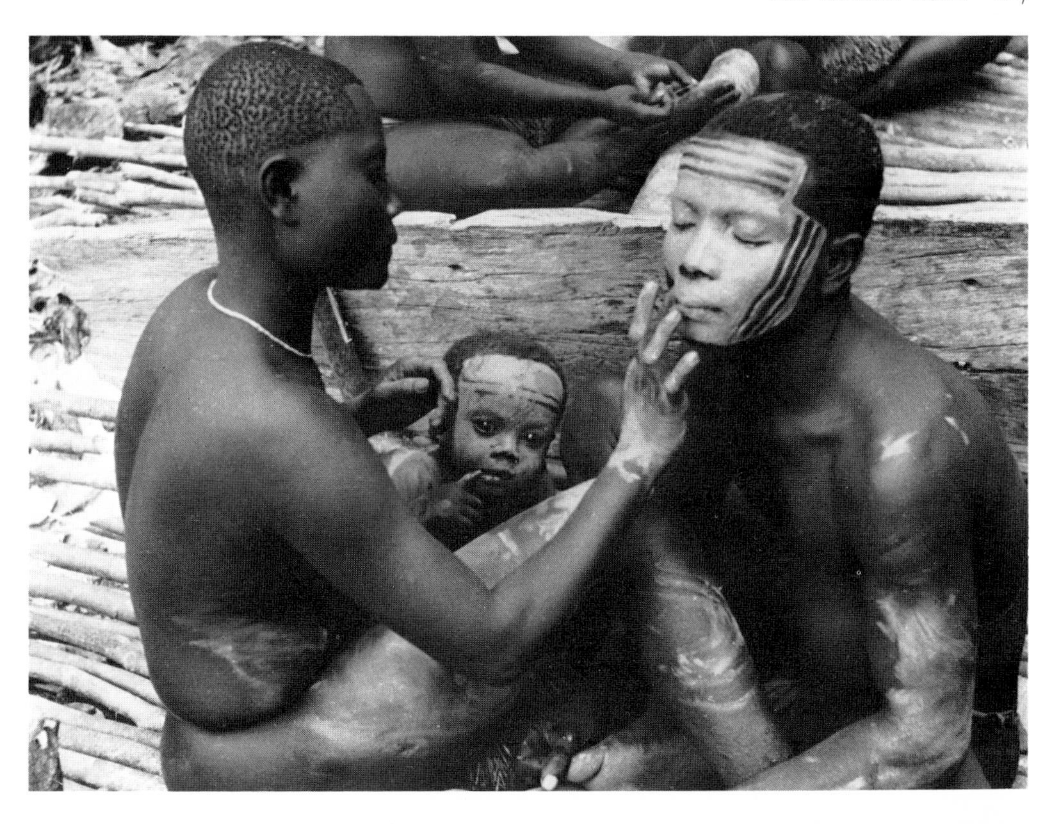

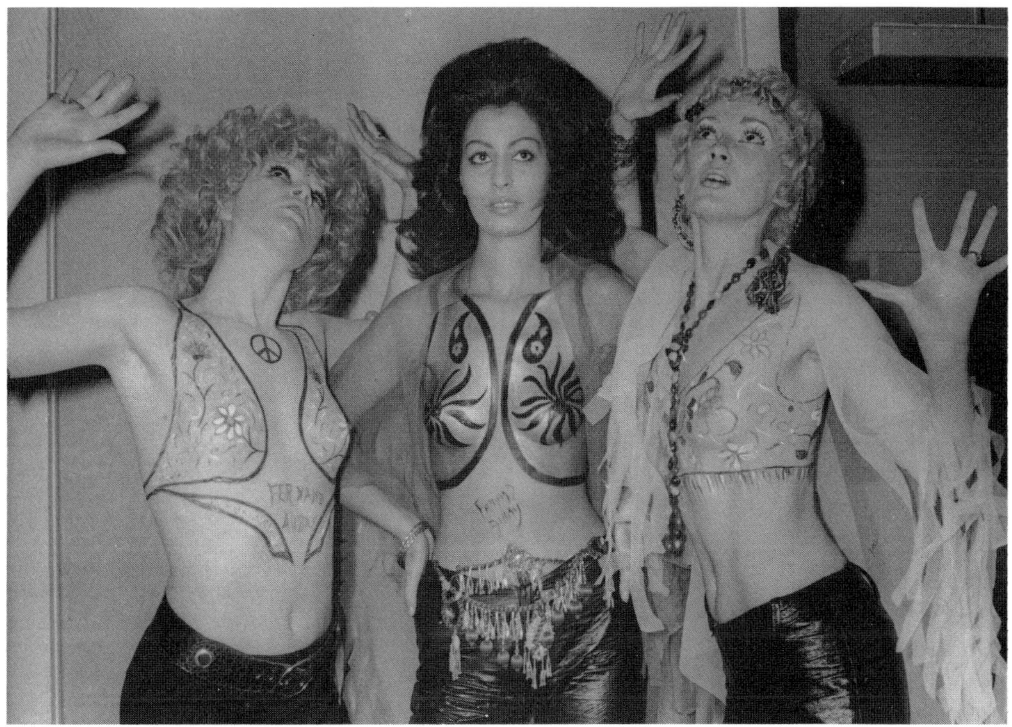

create a heightened sensual experience.

Whatever the deeper social or religious meaning behind body decoration, the sexual element rarely seems to be totally absent. As we have seen, Hagen body painting demonstrates relations between the living and the dead and conveys the cosmological beliefs of the community. But it also celebrates the attractive body, and at ceremonies and rites there is often an atmosphere of carnival. At dances and courting parties, in particular, individuals paint and ornament their bodies to impress members of the opposite sex. For courting parties, the men gather special leaves or grasses and put them in their hair, complementing their painted and charcoaled faces. Short trains of beads and cloths adorn the back of the girls' heads, and shell crescents are placed over their breasts. Their hair is oiled and their foreheads charcoaled and painted with a red band, while multicoloured spots and triangles are painted on their cheeks. They are said to mix love magic with their pigments and the men do the same with their grease. On their headdress the men wear a red flower of the *kila* tree; it is the brightness of these flowers which attracts flocks of birds and in the same way the Hageners aim to attract women. Bright red and fragrant, the flowers are a direct agent of sexual attraction. Their shape is supposed to give the whole male body a phallic form.

*A Dani (New Guinea) with penis sheath. The sheath, like tribal marks, may be used as a distinctive group sign.*

Paint, tattooing, ornaments and hairstyles accentuate the differences between the male and the female body. Differences between the human male and female bodies are not all that conspicuous: a man and a woman, naked, wearing the same ornaments and hairstyle, are very much alike. For this reason, we have invented distinctive male and female ornamentation, ways of walking and cosmetics; no society—apart from a recent unisex fashion in the West—dresses or decorates men and women in exactly the same way. (In this context, it is interesting that children often fail to distinguish the sexes when they are nude, only marking the difference when they put on skirts and trousers and little-boy and little-girl hairstyles.)

Among animals, on the other hand, sexual differentiation is often obvious.

> One of the greatest of sex allurements would be lost and the extreme importance of clothes would disappear at once if the two sexes were to dress alike; such identity of dress has never come about among any people. (Havelock Ellis)

pages 130 and 131 *Sexuality and beauty universally play a role in body decoration. The Fulani of West Africa have beauty contests for the boys. During these contests they submit to whipping while displaying an elaborately decorated body and painted face, with patterns in red and indigo. During the youths' beauty contest, the Fulani girls, loaded with bracelets, necklets and rings, watch the men, their indigo veils held together with finely worked chains and bead ropes.*

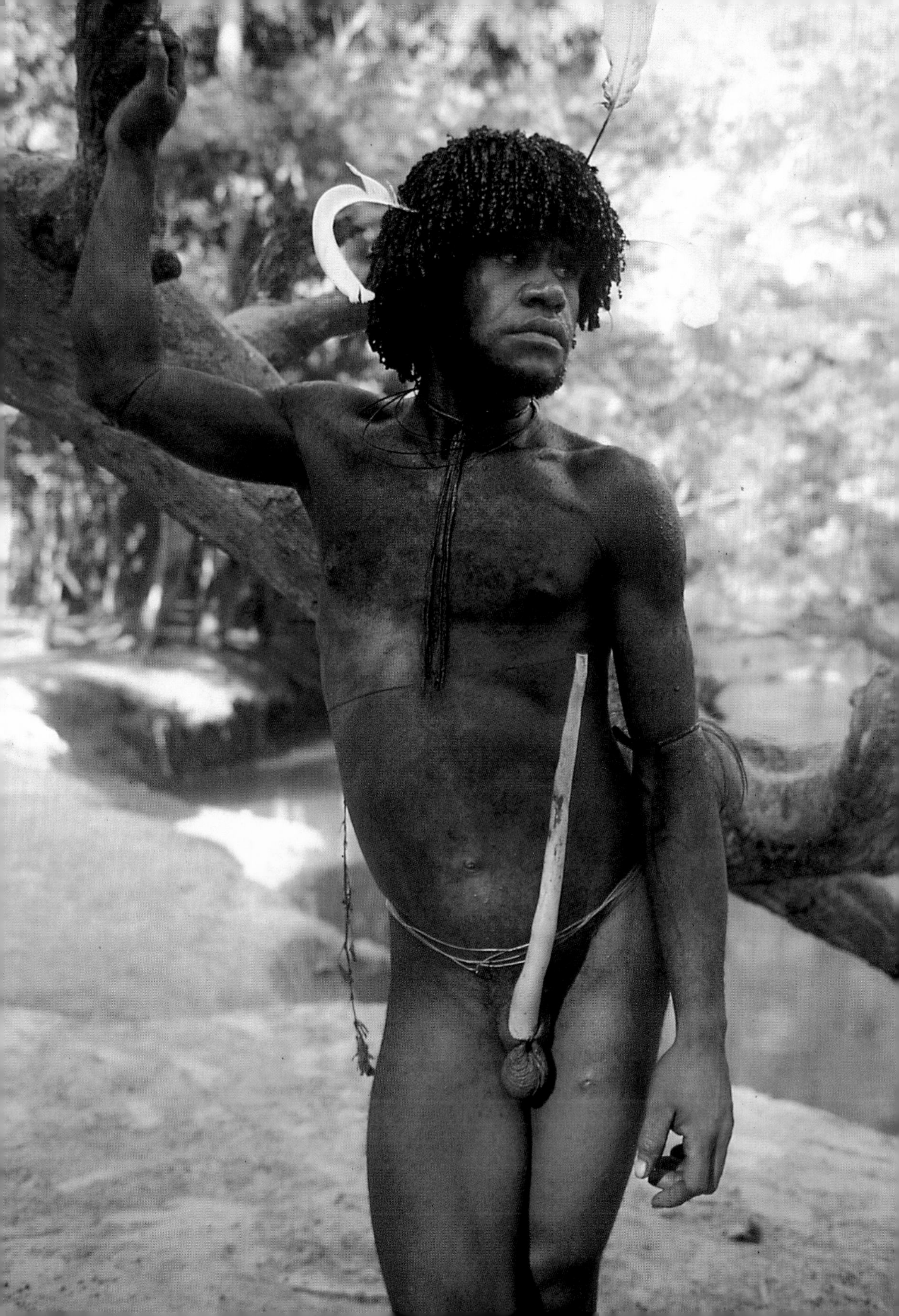

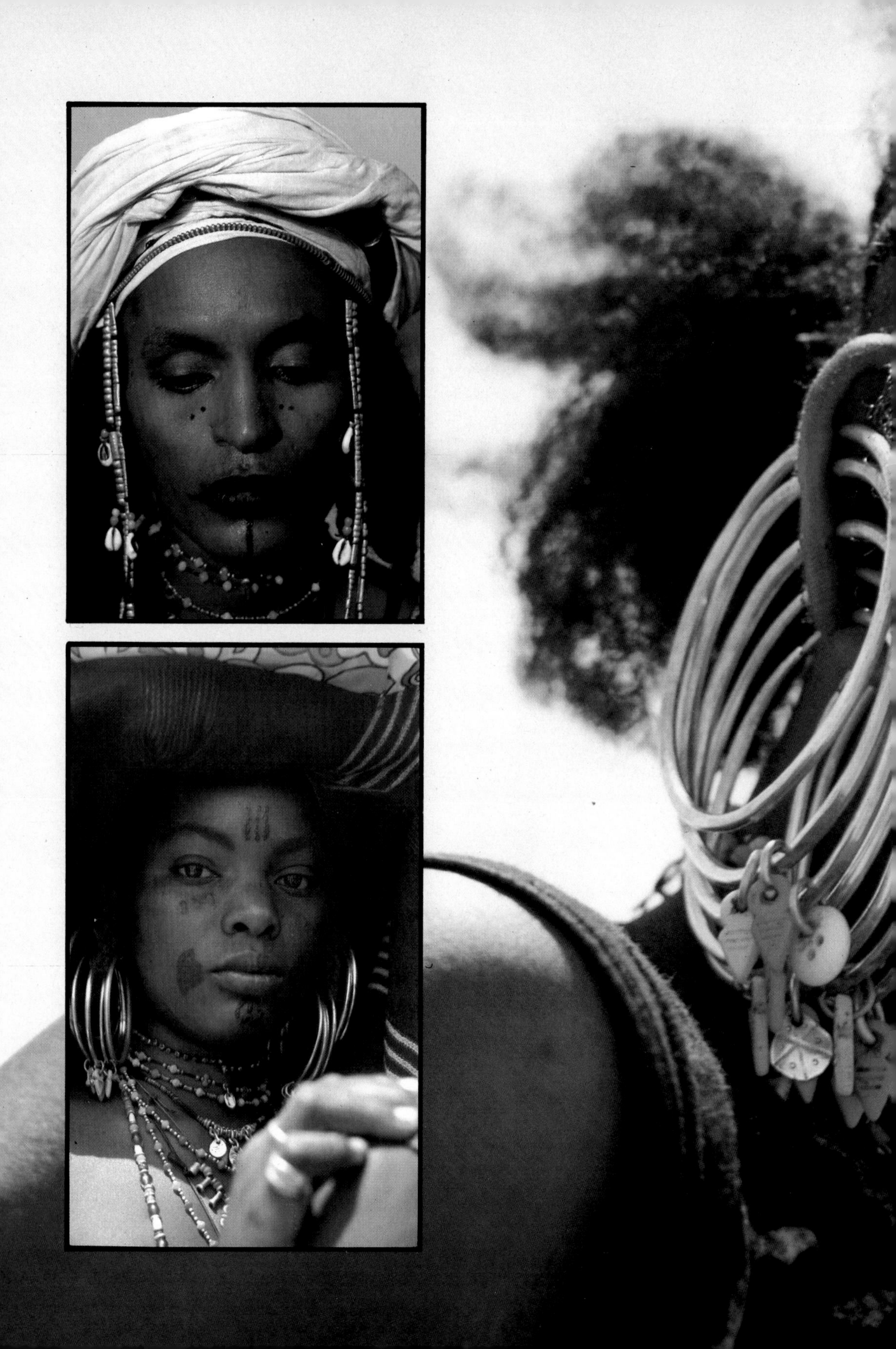

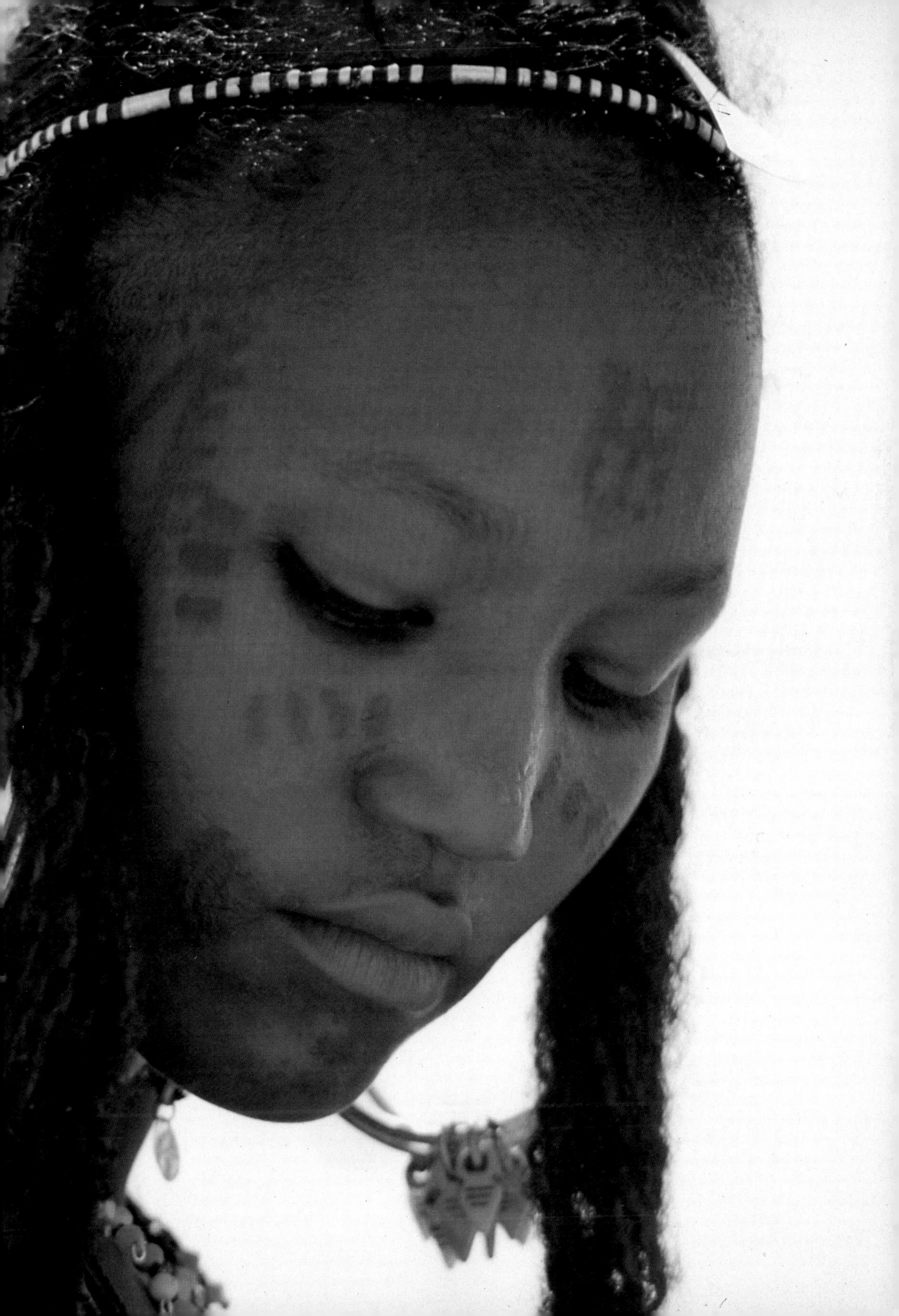

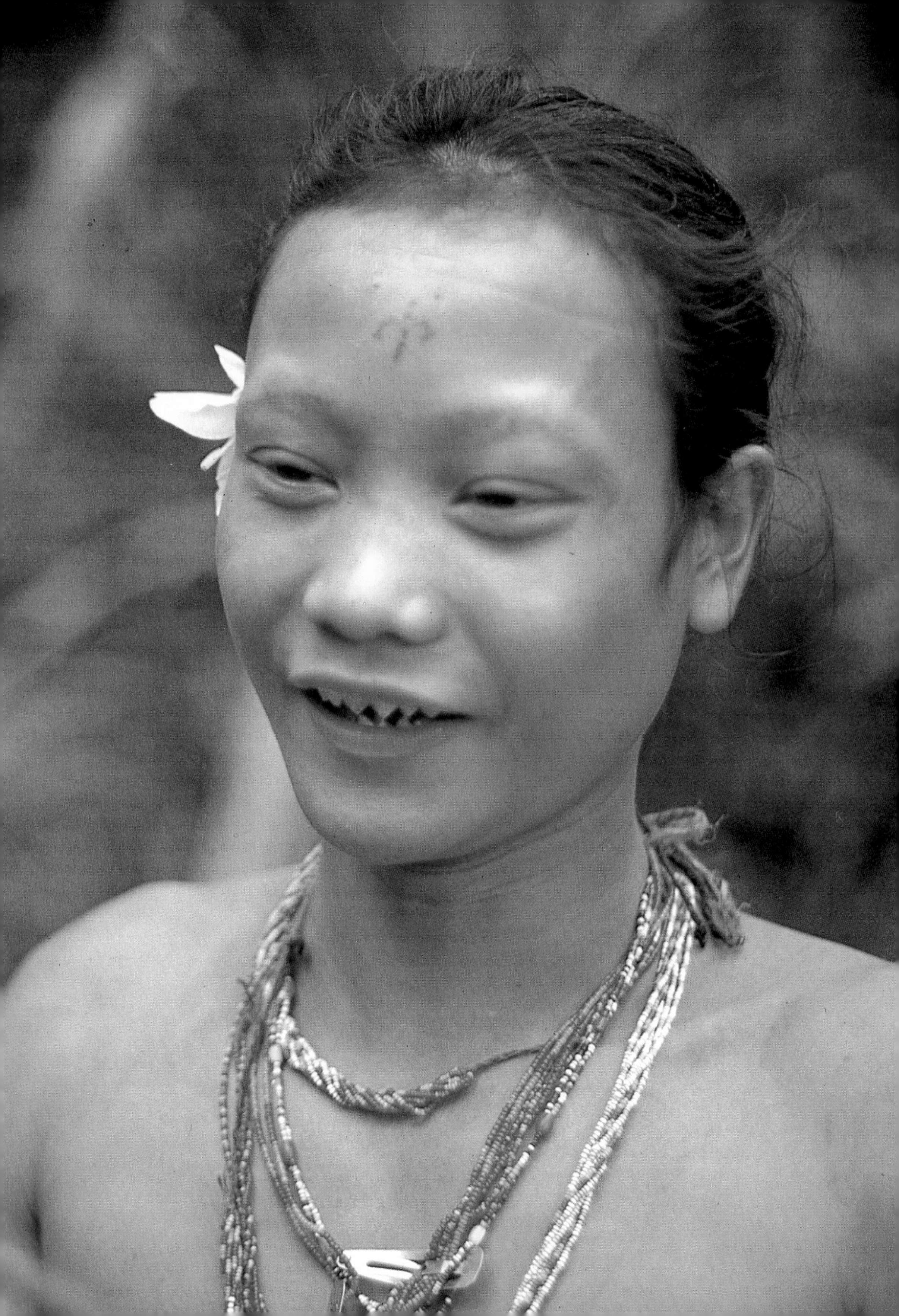

*Teeth are rarely left as nature intended them. Some peoples chip or file them in order to make them less like animal fangs, as with this young Mentawei Islander from Sumatra.*

And despite the unisex movement of the second half of the twentieth century, it is true that clothes, and perhaps more importantly body decoration, have served to accentuate sexual identity and attract the opposite sex.

The penis sheath, the great concealer of male genitalia, may serve as sexual display in the same way as the padded, decorated codpiece: each hides what it wishes to display, a man's masculinity. But even in the case of the penis sheath we cannot always be sure that it has phallic connotations. Sometimes it is a symbol of modesty. Sometimes, as for the Dani of New Guinea, the gourd sheath is used like tribal marks as a distinctive group sign: different communities are recognizable according to the length and width of the sheath and the angle at which it is held. We have already seen that the Suya, among whom the sheath is assumed at puberty, look on the object not as a symbol of sexual maturity but as a social control of that sexuality.

The Fulani care for their bodies from childhood, proud of their racial characteristics and determined to be beautiful as Fulani men or Fulani women. There are men's and women's ways of walking, sitting and talking; men's and women's ways of painting the body; men's and women's ways of ornamenting and fashioning hair into particular shapes and patterns. As far as the men are concerned, this differentiation is most marked during the *gerewol* male beauty contest when the most handsome and vain youths use all their arts of personal decoration to glorify themselves and the Fulani concept of male beauty. The ideal of Fulani male beauty is a clear pale skin, a slender body, supple and fine, a straight nose, a high forehead (which is shaven), smooth hair, a long neck, large eyes and white teeth.

During the *gerewol*, the boys are on show to the girls, who choose those who please them. One of the objectives of the male beauty contest is for a boy to get a wife, which reverses the trend in Western society. There are also tests of endurance, when a splendidly painted and adorned youth chooses a challenger to whip him. While he is beaten across his ochre-painted ribs, he expresses his virility and hence his sexuality by submitting without flinching, holding his arms above his head or languidly fingering a necklace while he gazes at his painted face in a mirror. Large weals result from this test and exhibition, and these are visible for life as raised ridges, and as among German duellists and some footballers these weals are highly prized as part of their body decoration.

*As well as tattooing their bodies for erotic purposes, the Japanese coloured their teeth, as Utamaro's print of a young woman at her toilet depicts.*

The Fulani girls watch their men. They are themselves loaded with bracelets, necklets and brass rings; their indigo veils, which cover their bodies, are held together with finely worked chains and bead ropes. The youths, oiled, ornamented and painted, line up before the women like red and indigo gods, their hair decorated with cowries and surmounted by long ostrich feathers. At each side of the face hang fringes of ram's beard, chains, beads and rings. Their faces are painted in red stripes, delicately bordered with indigo, and the same indigo paint is used to darken the lips. At the corners of the mouth are dark triangular patterns, while other designs are painted on the nose and cheeks. The basic complexion colour is ochre, and the upper half of the body, the chest and the neck, is polished like mahogany. Each youth also carries a ceremonial axe, the crest of which represents a man's coiffure while the patterns of the body painting are worked on it.

The *gerewol* ceremony and its display of male sexuality and beauty lasts seven days. The young men are decorated as the future stud bulls of this nomadic community. The festival begins with a prayer-like chant. The young men line up, singing the same weird high note and balance lightly on the balls of their feet, looking ahead at the women. They hold themselves straight, arms linked, baring their eyes and teeth. The whole crowd comments and criticizes, old ladies making fun of the ugly and ungainly. The boys continue to make *mous*, arching their bodies and rolling their eyes as the girls come towards them and kneel in front of them. A girl leaves the group and approaches them, the boys frantically preening and making faces in an effort to seduce her and choose them. With a slight movement of the arm she indicates the dancer she has chosen.

Of course, the 'sexual' explanation of cosmetics is as one-sided and reductionist as the 'magical' explanation. If sexuality or magic are given as prime motives behind body painting or tattooing, this is often due to the interest or prejudice of the ethnographer. The Andaman Islanders are an example. For instance, Radliffe-Brown stresses the social context of body painting. We have already pointed out that among these islanders body painting seems to be an art for art's sake. Cipriani sees only vanity and sexuality, and according to him the care with which the Andamaners paint their bodies is due to the desire to attract the opposite sex: 'the more a wife loves her husband' the more magnificent the designs she executes

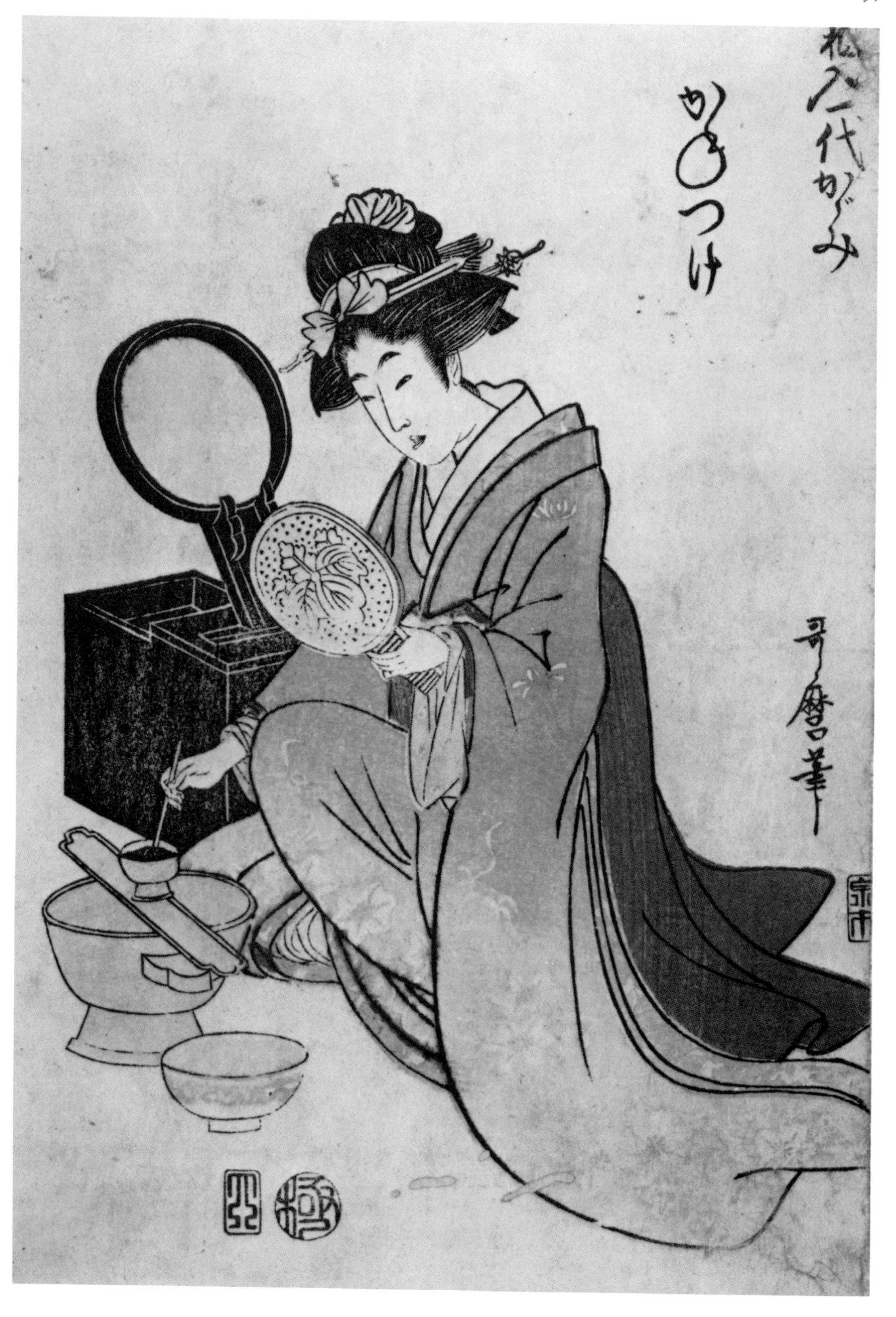
哥麿筆

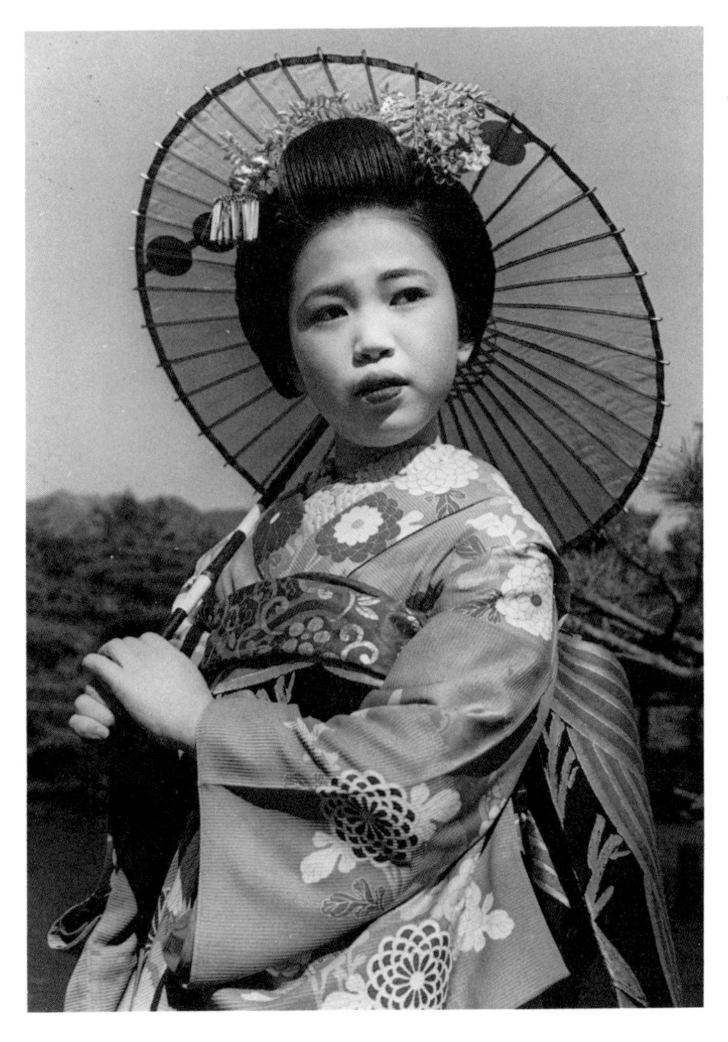

*Body painting is only one of the techniques of seduction. A sixteen-year-old Japanese student geisha must learn all the body arts, including gesture and deportment.*

for him. Yet despite his insistence on sexuality, his statements contradict him: 'The paintings on their bodies reach a peak every two or three days as they fear illness and death if they are not newly daubed.' A man returning from a successful hunting trip is met by his wife who executes exceptionally elaborate designs; they also paint their most interesting and significant designs after the colossal feasts which follow a big hunt.

In the West, we are used to associating make-up with vanity and sexuality. Clothes and make-up and cosmetic surgery accentuate women's erogenous zones: the corset narrows the waist, enhances the abdominal and gluteal regions and pushes up the breasts. Thus women exaggerate their female characteristics. Their hairstyles are usually large, making the face look smaller; bare white breasts and pale clothes, particularly around the throat, give a feminine look which contrasts with the dark hairy jaws and hairy chest of the male. Cosmetics are often painfully sexual in inspiration, hardly less subtle than the bright natural colours of the baboon during oestrus. The female mouth is given an intense sexual significance with the red slash of lipstick, a violent display of femininity, although sometimes attention is taken away from the mouth, and the eyes become the centre of the face. A woman's eyelashes are longer and stronger than a man's, making the eyes themselves look larger. The thinner more delicate tissues surrounding a woman's eyes are responsive to changes in mood and emit strong signals, which are accentuated by mascara and dark eye cosmetics. Belladonna, dropped into the eyes, enlarges the pupil, robbing the eye for a time of its natural protection against bright light and increasing its brilliance. Dark eyes for women are often associated with a pale, passive complexion, achieved by devices such as pancake make-up, which reduces facial movement and enhances the impression of femininity.

Make-up is 'man-proof' and marketed under such names as *Sin* and *Scandal*. However, it is obvious that cosmetics need not express a blatant sexuality to be sold. Youthfulness and social approval are important, especially for older women.

Western ornamentation may have more complex and subtle associations, concerned with conforming to an image and reflecting the fundamental values of society. It may even reflect the opposite of sexuality, calling attention to the face as a way of denying strong urges linked with another part and drawing attention away from the genital area.

On the whole, make-up and cosmetic surgery demonstrate the Western people's devotion to fashion, their passion for conformity rather than sexuality. Women cover themselves with make-up, wearing their mask even when their lovers declare a hatred of paints and powders. Husbands who adore large breasts often lose them to the cosmetic surgeon. In the United States, it is even possible for a cosmetician to suggest that balding should be cured by castration, which would bring back the disappearing hair.

The strongest motivation in cosmetic sales does, in fact, seem to be the pursuit of social, not sexual, satisfaction.

*chapter eight*

# The Animal Body

*Man from north-west Kenya decorated for a ceremony. The painting and lip plug have special significance, while the symbolism of the bush—the ostrich feathers and leopard-skin cloak—add further essential elements to his costume.*

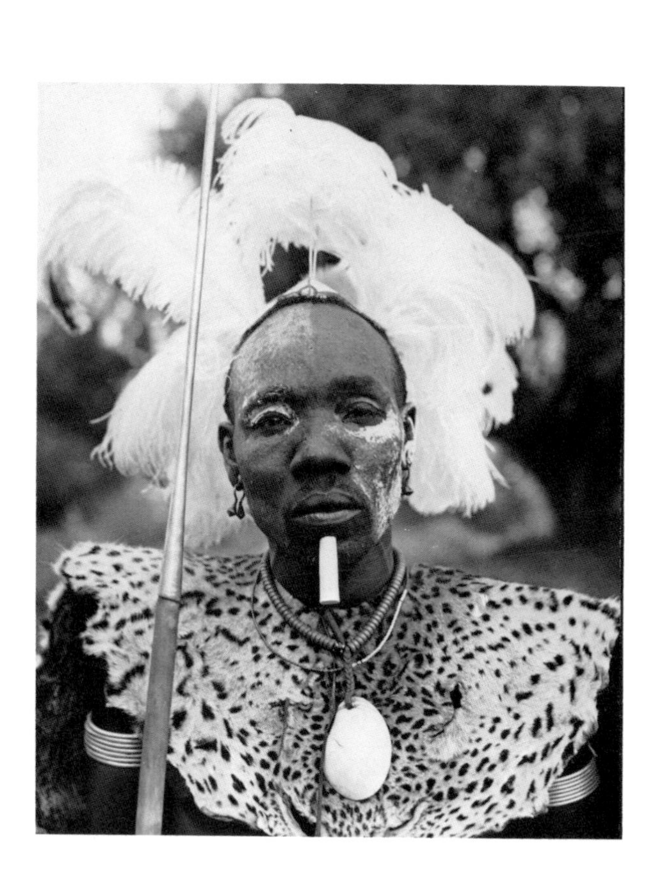

MANY NINETEENTH-CENTURY theorists believed that primitive men daubed or cut their bodies as lustful animals. Even in the present century some writers have assumed that body decoration is in some way a kind of mimicry of nature. They have attributed body painting to an attempt by humans to resemble the animals among which they live. The notion was that primitive peoples put on 'protective coloration', adapting to the prevalent hues of their environment, or 'warning coloration', as a sign of aggression. In the former, they camouflaged their bodies like animals which harmonize with a predominant colour scheme, and it has been pointed out that the mottled, disruptive, grey-green pattern used in modern battledress closely resembles that of cryptically coloured animals. However, in most societies war usually brings out 'warning coloration' rather than 'protective coloration'. Before the nineteenth century, in the West and elsewhere, warriors wore distinctive bright patterns or tattooed themselves, like the Maori in their *moko* designs, to be conspicuous and frightening.

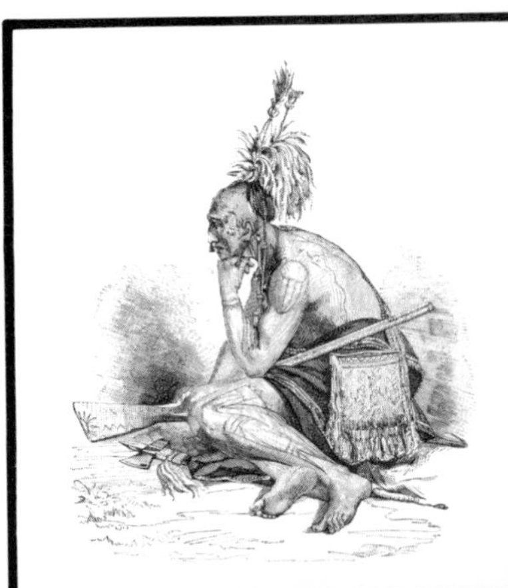

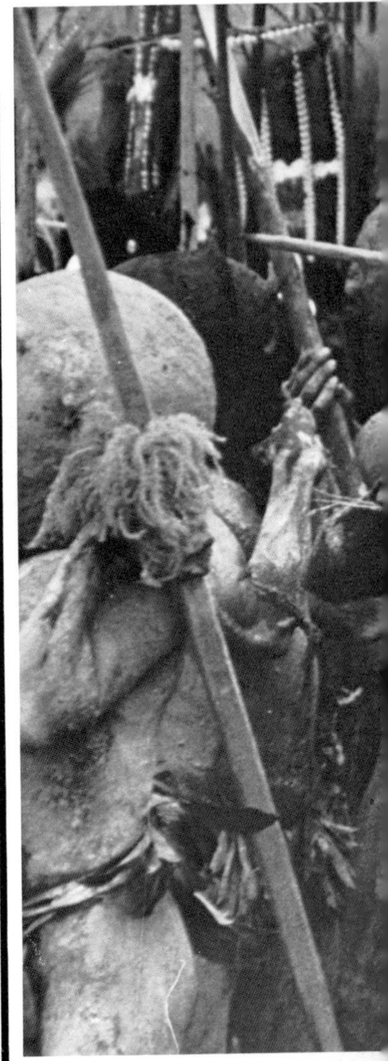

Hunting peoples assumed 'protective coloration' for practical purposes. Australians evaded detection when stalking game by covering their bodies with red ochre, earth or clay. Kangaroo hunters disguised themselves with blue earth in the blue mud flats and with red ochre in the laterite zones. Bushmen hunters, in Africa, achieved camouflage by posture, movement, sound and paint. They painted themselves with red and yellow stripes in imitation of the zebra. They swayed like the animal, made animal noises or remained perfectly still. When stalking ostriches they used an ostrich disguise, carrying the head of one of these birds on a long pliant stick, which they manipulated in suitable ways, keeping their bodies concealed. In North America, the Indians clothed themselves in a wolf skin and moved like a wolf when approaching a herd of bison, for bison had no fear of a solitary wolf.

However, it is a mistake to assume animal mimicry in all body decoration. Among the Coniagui of Guinea, as among the Galliacea, the privilege of wearing immense crests in the shape of cockscombs is reserved for young men, as a symbol of potency (at least this is the explanation of the ethnographer). Others point to the sexual display of groups which put on stags' horns or the heavy mane of a bison, implying that they are imitating the male animal in his splendour before the female. As we have seen, the Fulani dress up sumptuously and dance like peacocks in front of the young girls. One observer likened the *gerewol* ceremony to the mating dance of birds;

left *In war many peoples, like this Canadian Indian, paint in bright and gaudy fashion, with the intention of intimidation. It might also ensure good luck.* below *The masked dances of these New Guinea warriors were once performed as a prelude to war. Now these mud decorations form part of a ceremonial dance of the people of the Asaro River.*

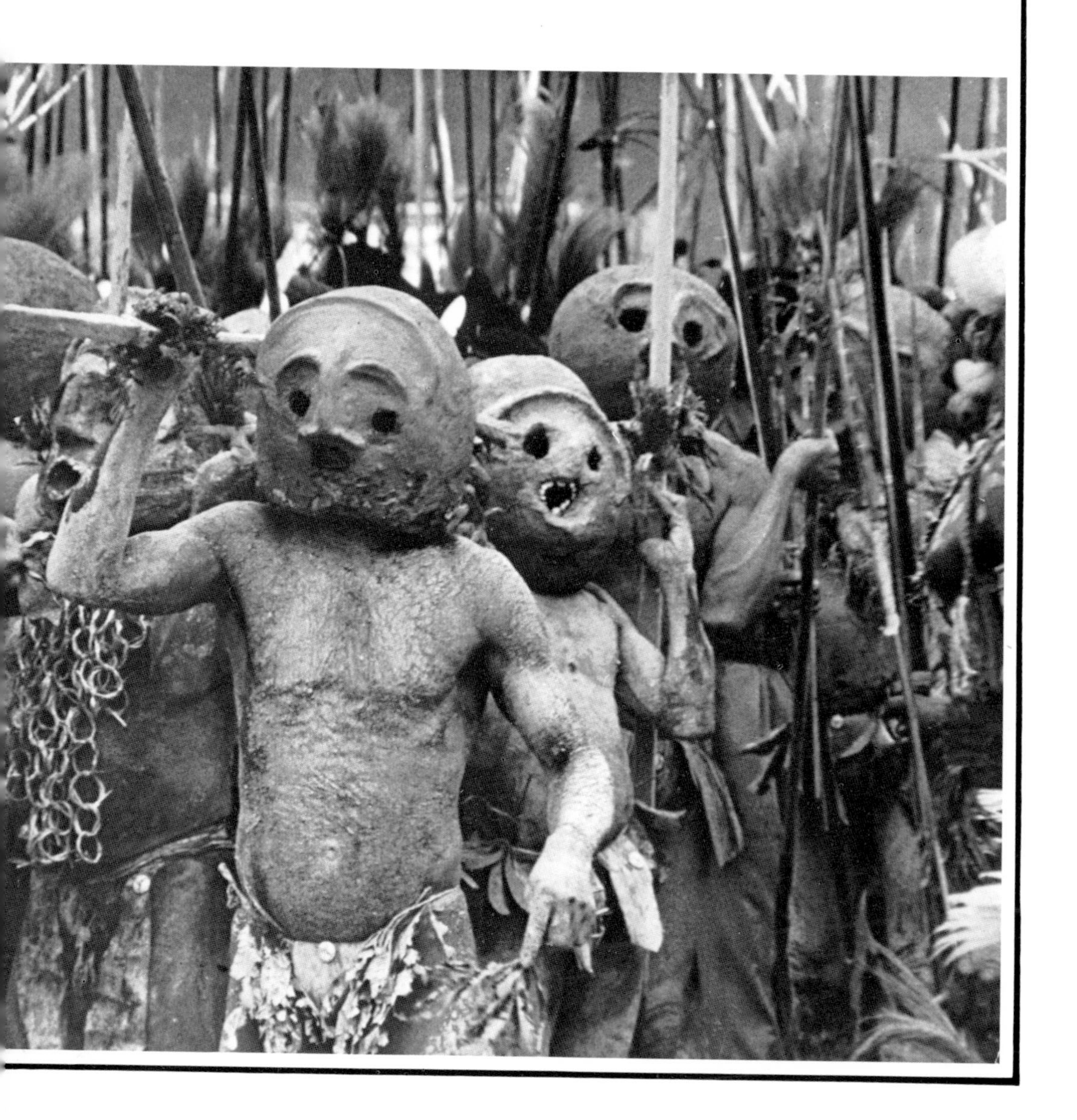

another compared the parade of young men before the nubile girls to the rivalry among their cattle herds during the mating season; but we have already noted that Fulani beauty competitions reflect not animal lust but a display of ideal male beauty in a race-conscious society.

In war, men painted themselves in bright and gaudy fashion, in colours which had aggressive, intimidating connotations. Our own soldiers, before the development of modern weapons and tactics, wore bright colours, often red, to overawe the enemy (and also to conceal the extent of their wounds). The ceremonial uniforms of the American Marines, the French Paras, the British Brigade of Guards, and the elaborate uniforms of the Spanish and Italian police are relics of this. The adornment of the American Indian in war paint was intended to frighten the enemy, not hide the attacker. Red has always been a popular colour for soldiers; 'Redskins' were so called from the colour of their paint. In Ancient Rome, victorious leaders were carried in triumph to the Capitol, their faces and chests painted red.

But even painting for war is not necessarily straightforward aggression. In Gran Chaco in South America, the Indians painted the face and body and ornamented themselves with rhea plumes to ensure good luck and supernatural protection. Rather differently, when a Jibaro warrior returned from battle he painted his body black as a protection against the soul of the slain enemy. Black, as we have already seen, was used by the Thompson Indians when they killed enemies or important animals *out of respect for the dead.* Paint consecrated the warrior who had killed or who was about to kill, protecting him from supernatural dangers associated with taking human life. An Aranda Australian would paint his face and body in bright colours if he had killed during a raid, and would not talk for a period. Among the Motu of New Guinea, it was the victim who was painted in particular circumstances, for if they decided to give up a murderer—rather than engaging in a blood feud—the man retired to his house where he ornamented and painted himself. When day dawned, the murderer descended the ladder of his house and was speared to death by his enemies.

Brightly marked animals use their coloration for camouflage, warning, sexual display and so on—in fact for reasons similar to those used by humans, and sometimes coloration which was apparently originally designed for one purpose is adapted for another. Normally the function of the swollen perianal region in sexually receptive female primates is a sign of sexual availability. The female baboon presents her backside with the tail up or to one side as an invitation to the male to mate. But this behaviour pattern is also used to inhibit aggression from other members of the group, of either sex, and is used as a kind of greeting to any higher ranking individuals. The swelling and coloration of the backside is particularly conspicuous in those species which have the most aggressive and quarrelsome males. Males will do the same, not of course as an invitation to mate but to inhibit aggression, presenting their bright bottoms to males higher in the pecking order.

The temptation to make comparisons between animal and human behaviour in cases like this is great and in both animals and man, whatever the original purpose of a natural or artificial adornment, it may be adapted in time to suit quite different needs. The smile, for example, has its instinctive physiological precursor, but this in no way contradicts the fact that the social form of the smile has become a language in its own right, with different meanings in Japan and America, regulated by social rules and conventions.

Notwithstanding this, zoologists such as Konrad Lorenz and Desmond Morris, have maintained that cosmetics are *sexual* triggers, manifestations of inborn patterns which we share with animals. For them, animal coloration and human make-up is embedded in the complex of human behaviour necessary for the continuation of the human species, and the urge to make up is induced by the same elementary force that serves the continuation of the species.

Darwin has already stressed the importance of colour and bright beauty in sexual selection. Plants glow, awaiting insects to fertilize them; insects, such as the firefly, make a wild effort to shine for their moment of ephemeral union. The male mandrill has a bright red penis with blue scrotal patches on either side, and the colour pattern is repeated on the face—its nose is bright red and its swollen, naked cheeks an intense blue, the animal's face mimicking its genital region. These animal facts gave Desmond Morris the idea that our vertical posture and frontal sexual position has resulted in most of our sexual signals and erogenous zones being placed on the front of our bodies, the protuberant, hemispherical breasts of the female being copies of the fleshy buttocks, and the sharply defined lips copies of the red labia. However, such comparisons are glib. Among humans, many sexual attributes become div-

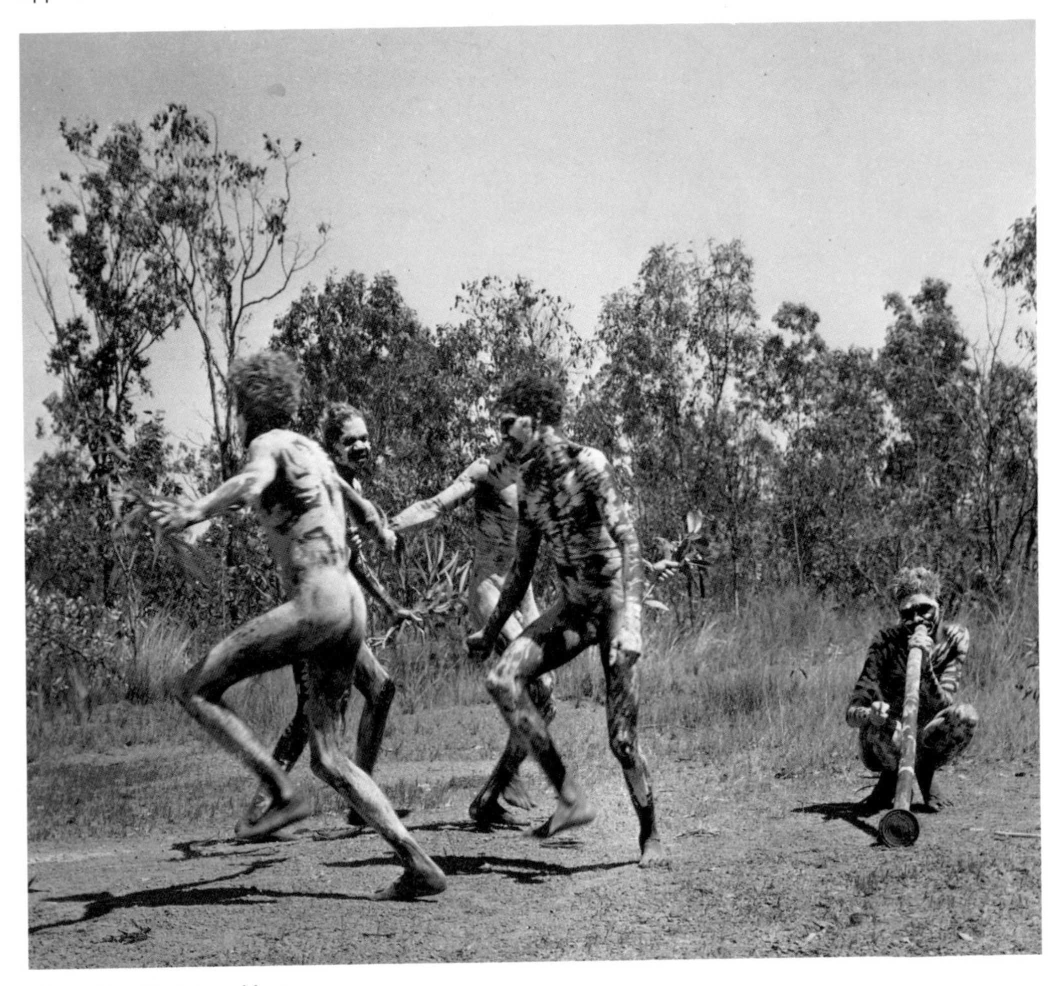

*Australian Aborigines celebrate totemic spirits in their dances and ceremonies. Men painted with ochre imitate the movements of the Australian crane, the brolga, to the accompaniment of the didgeridoo.*

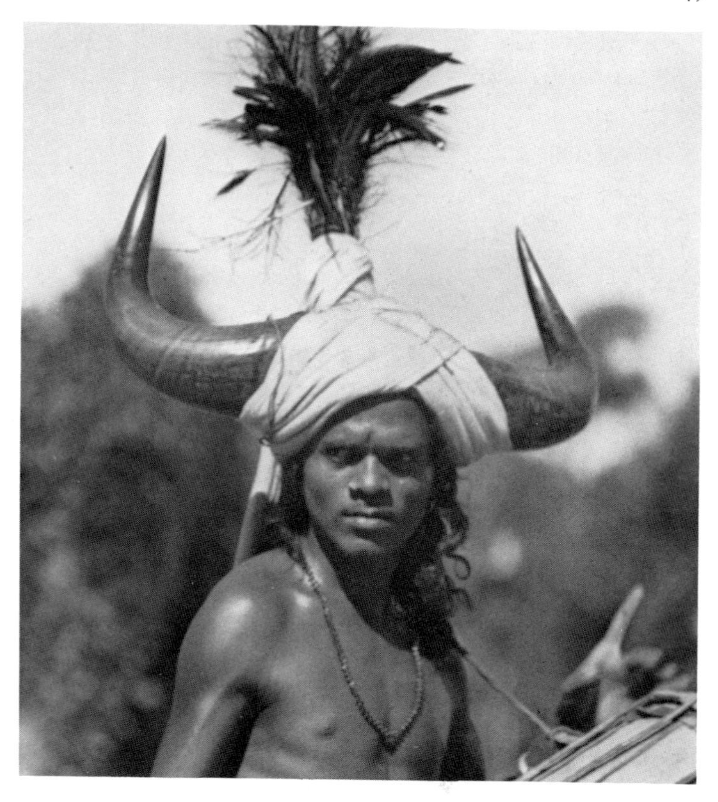

*A Gond from India demonstrates by his headdress his society's symbolic relationship with the bison.*

orced from their original context. Women in the West wear make-up which is blatantly sexual, but they are not communicating their sexual availability, they are merely following fashion.

Bright colours, then, in humans, animals and birds are not exclusively sexual in purpose, and in some cases colour only secondarily attracts the female. It may be significant that in polygynous species like the moose, the seal and the elephant, the head of the group is a supermale in terms of display, size and adornment, while in monogamous species, like the coyote and the wolf, male and female are similar. In the case of Western peoples, among monogamous couples it is the female who today wears bright cosmetics and marks of distinction, and austerity in male dress (apart from some religious groups) has been a twentieth-century phenomenon. We might well ask why women in a monogamous Christian society are so gaudily displayed, when church and state and general morals have always attempted to prevent them mating with men other than their husbands.

I would suggest that the motivation behind body art is not derived from animals but is purely human. We can find no one-to-one relationship between animal coloration and the countless different ways in which men and women adorn their bodies. In a specifically practical, hunting situation, as in Australia, men may mimic animals, but in their ceremonies in honour of totemic spirits, abstract, geometric designs are employed.

Cosmetics, in fact, separate us from the animal world. The Bathonga in Africa declare that their bodies are scarified to distinguish them from fish. People who file their teeth say they do it to differentiate themselves from animals with undecorated teeth. Painted bodies serve to emphasize the difference between men and animals. All human societies use body decoration to disguise their kinship with animals; clothing, ornaments and painting attempt to underline man's kinship with the world of culture, not the world of nature, with the gods and the spirits, not the animals. Decoration distinguishes us from the brutes.

That most people prefer to forget their animal nature was shown in 1859 when the Victorian world greeted with rage and disgust the publication of Darwin's epoch-making *On the Origin of Species*, with its theory that man was not a special creature of divine interposition.

Man wants to display his 'cultural' human qualities, not his 'natural' beastly attributes. Body hair is an example. Many peoples prefer to remove hair on the body to distinguish themselves from brute creation. Depilation is a form of body decoration found all over the world; the face, the eyebrows, the pubic regions and the legs are the parts most subjected to this practice. The numerous advertisements for depilatories and the curious popularity of the shaven face demonstrate our desire to look unlike animals.

The Egyptians shaved off their body hair using depilatory creams, razors and pumice stones. Julius Caesar had his facial hair plucked out with tweezers and shaved himself all over, particularly before sex. The Roman poet Ovid, advising women in his *Ars Amatoria*, told them to 'let no rude goat find his way beneath your arms and let not your legs be rough with bristling hair.' Hindus believe they are more desirable without body hair. Even Australians consider that a handsome man is a man with no body hair except on the head and face, and spend hours plucking and shaving superfluous hair. The facts seem odd: we go to extremes to remove natural hair, yet pubic hair and armpit and body hair are natural sexual stimulants and grow in areas where the skin contains scent glands. Pubic hair is a scented recognition signal and a stimulant to sexual excitement—yet we shave it off. The reason is clear: a hairy body is an animal body. Wild men, like Esau the hunter, are hairy. Body hair is beastly and has to go in the interests of humanity.

*chapter nine*

# The Social Body

*Once upon a time, wig shapes set professional groups apart and came to be associated with medical, legal or military professions. Today, in some parts of the world, lawyers and judges still wear distinctive wigs dating from the eighteenth century. The inset photograph is of an English circuit judge. Around him are a selection of eighteenth-century wigs illustrated in Diderot's Encyclopedia.*

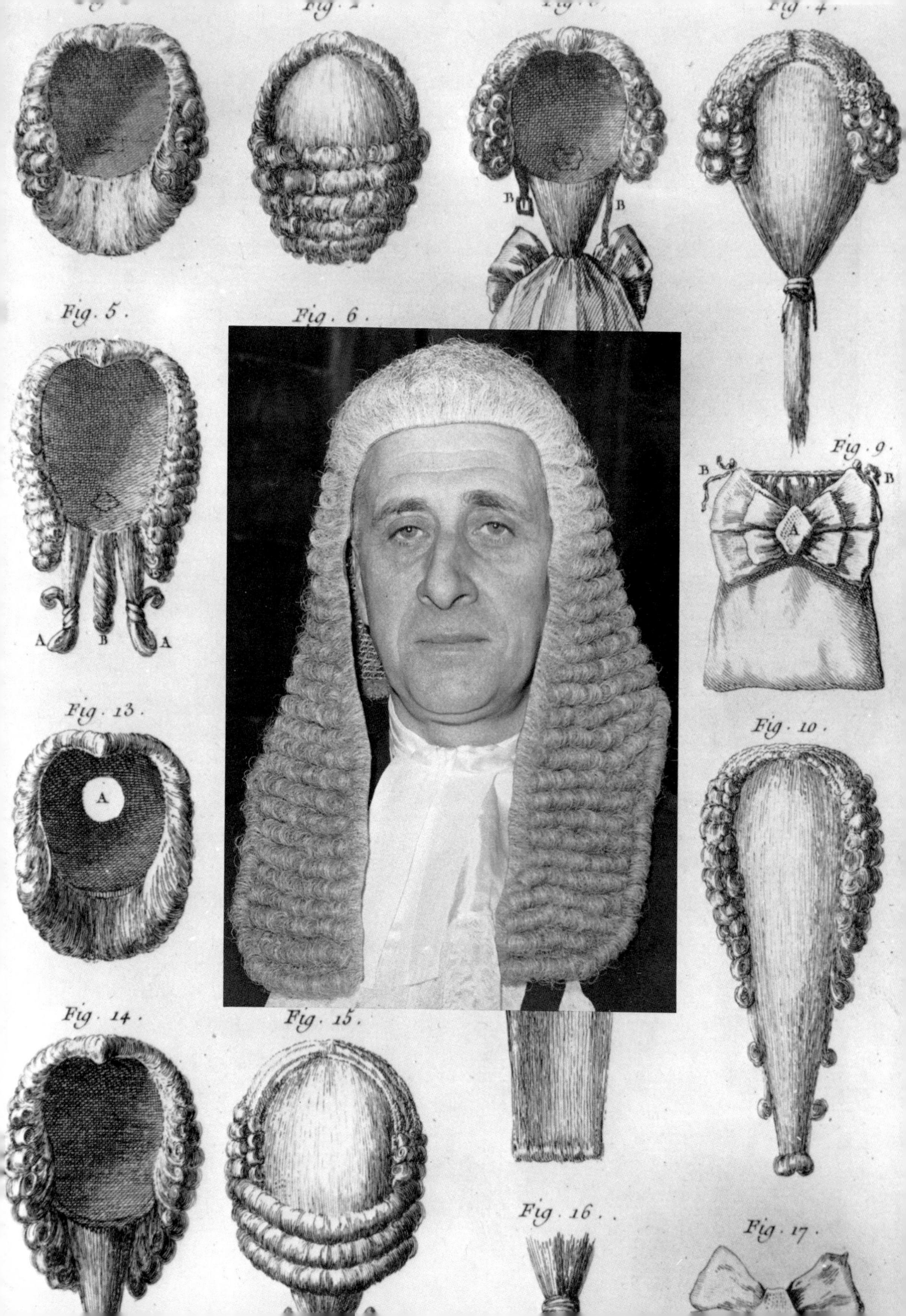
Fig. 4.
Fig. 5.
Fig. 6.
Fig. 9.
Fig. 10.
Fig. 13.
Fig. 14.
Fig. 15.
Fig. 16.
Fig. 17.

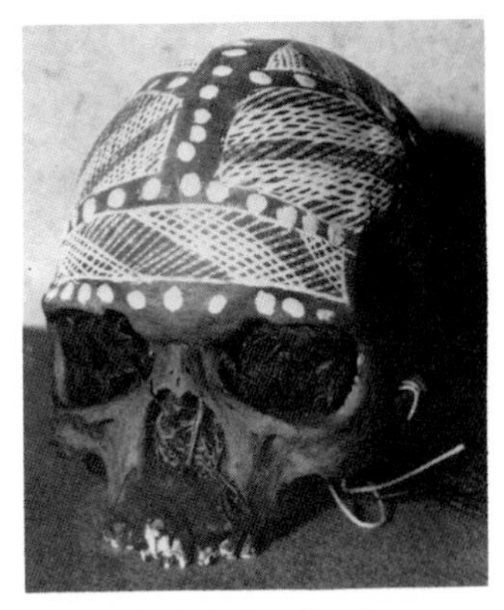

*The skulls of Arnhem Land Aborigines are painted with the same designs worn by dancers, designs which relate to the dead man's clan and myths. On this one the pattern signifies a muddy, weedy swamp, with bubbles rising to the surface.*

BODY PAINTING reflects the facts of social organization, as well as individual vanity, sexuality and business ambition. Body signs in ornaments, tattoos and clothes often serve as markers to separate groups or clans from each other. The symbols often express a sentiment of *esprit de corps*. When missionaries and administrators banned certain styles of body decoration, the loss to a society was almost as serious as the loss of a verbal language. In this way, conquerors undermine subordinate cultures. Thus the English forbad the wearing of the kilt, long hair and the Gaelic language in their attempt to subdue the Scottish Highlands. In the Pacific and Africa, they dressed conquered peoples in European clothes, covering up the tattoos, taught them the advantages of a short haircut and a neat parting, and made them learn about the Western world in the language of the colonizers.

Tattoos, scarification and painting may all provide signs of group belonging. In Hindu society, each Brahmin sub-caste had its own particular style of body-painting, usually an arrangement of lines, dashes or circles on the forehead, cheeks and chest; the followers of Siva and Vishnu had special signs.

During the dances and ceremonies in Arnhem Land, Australia, the designs painted on the participants demonstrate their membership of a particular kinship or language group. The designs, which are painted on the body with small brushes of human hair, are generally of sacred origin, being conventionalized representations of the clan country and its mythology. The patterns are the sole property of members of the clan, each individual possessing a number of distinctive designs on the same theme. The designs are commonly inherited from the father, but a person may gain the right to use the clan patterns of his mother's or his mother's mother's group in which he has subsidiary rights. His hereditary clan design, however, is of the greatest importance and he is careful of the use made of it and the attitude towards it, for it represents part of his spirit. Many of the blood feuds of the past were the result of a mark of disrespect towards a clan's designs or the theft of a pattern.

Arnhem Land designs, which are derived from ancestral or totemic beings, may be bartered or sold or exchanged, and incorporated in the patterns of other clans; and although traditional designs have often been altered by individual artists to suit special purposes, the old totemic pattern is retained and incorporated in the new. The exchange of clan designs is a give and take arrangement so that an individual may secure a

top right *The painted patterns on these Arnhem Land dancers are the sole property of the members of the clan and are inherited, though some patterns may be bartered, sold or exchanged.* right *Short hair or no hair is often a sign of submission to a higher authority. In a monastery in Taipeh, Buddhist monks are saying grace.*

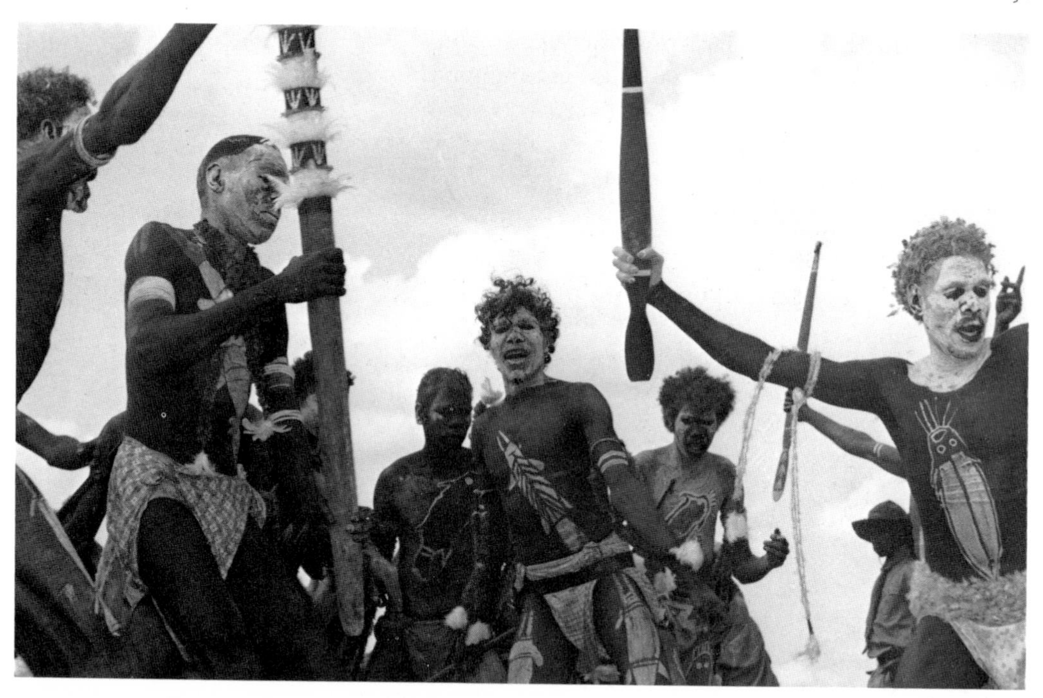

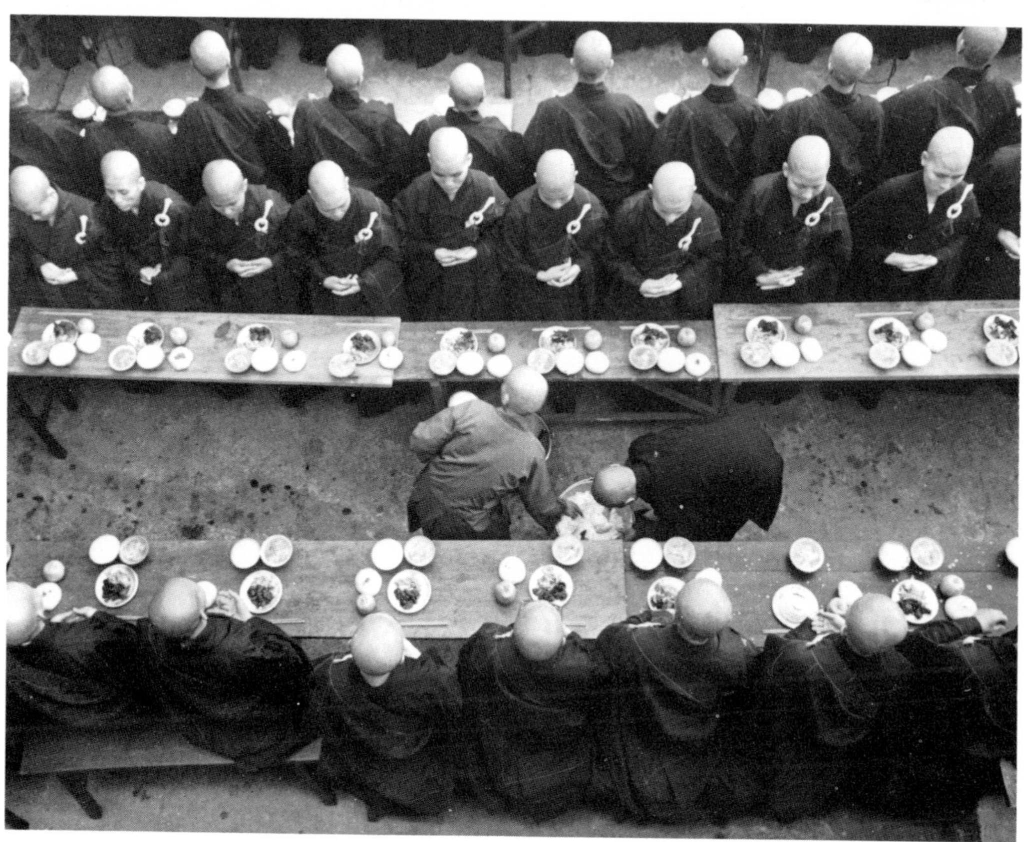

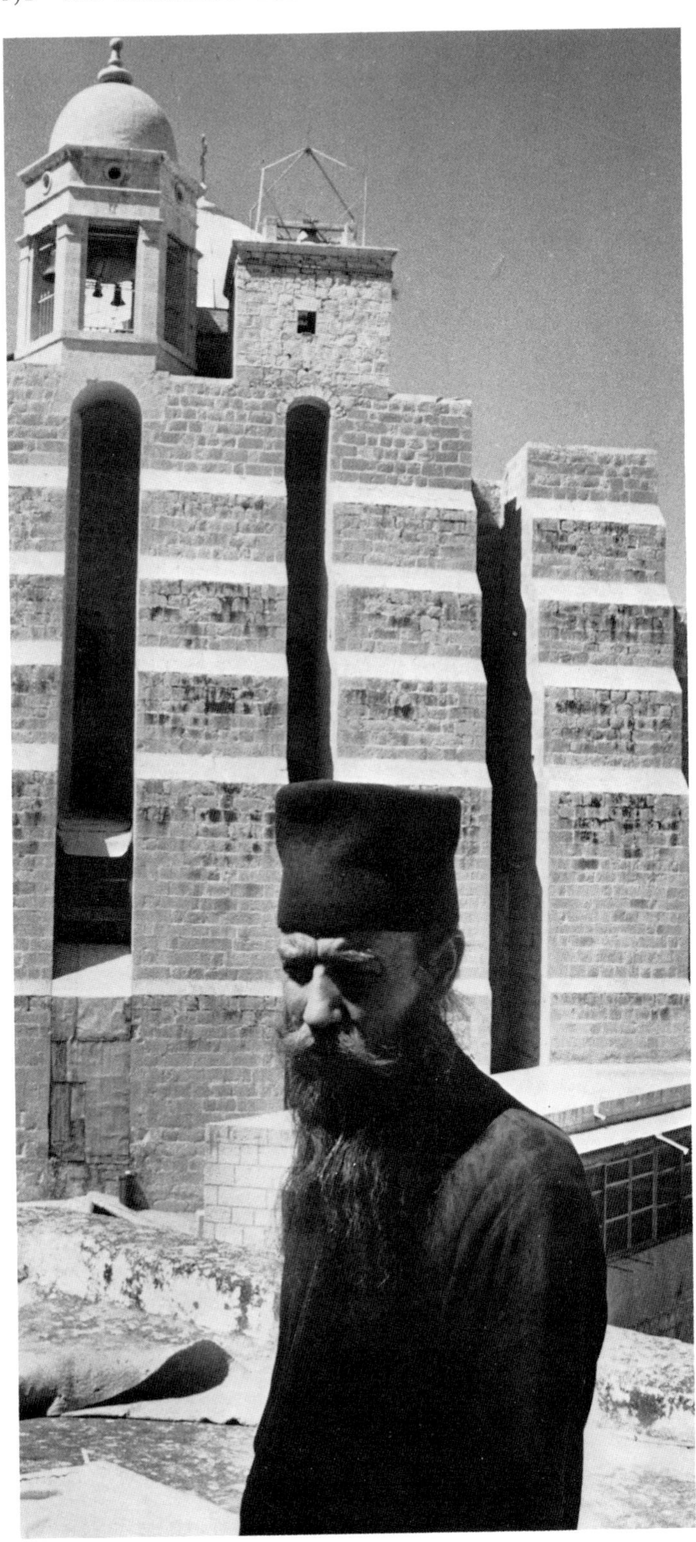

*While Buddhist monks shave their heads and many Christian monks are tonsured, this Russian-born Yugoslav monk at the Mar Sabba monastery in the Judean desert wears hair and beard long as a sign of his dedication.*

little of the spiritual force of the totems of all the clans in his territory. The exchange both symbolizes the differences between the clans and at the same time emphasizes the fact that the people are all united in a larger group.

Among the Arnhem Land Australians, then, the designs represent clans, and apart from their ritual uses also serve as a means of obtaining food and goods. Karel Kupka wrote in *Art in Arnhem Land:*

> Thus, a man may tell a friend that he will reveal to him, by painting his body, his own sacred totemic design. The friend cannot refuse. They go either to a secluded and temporarily sacred place, usually at one end of the main camp behind bushes, or to the secret ceremonial ground, or to a clearing in the adjacent bush. Here the friend is painted with the clan design of the artist, after which he may be 'sung' over. Later on he must 'pay' for the painting, for this is regarded as a sacred revelation like a totemic rite. The artist may paint several persons at the same time, and it is not unusual to see several artists at work in this way, with their subjects stretched out before them. The men, too, who carry out the painting, may themselves, in turn, be painted by others, and so incur obligations. Consequently, in due course, a man will have had the patterns of nearly all the clans painted on his chest, and will have 'paid' for them in food and goods.

Even in our own society we assert our special group affiliations by hairstyle, clothes and body markings, in the same way as people wear red rosettes for political Labour reasons or Gay Lib badges to express common corporate belonging rather than individual distinction. Hairstyles may reflect class or membership of youth groups, such as the mods and rockers, hippies and skinheads. Beard styles once reflected political currents. The Emperor Franz Josef's beard, the twirled, upturned ends of the Kaiser's moustache, the Italian Garibaldi beard, the Balbo beard of the Fascists and the brushed-up, stove-pipe hairstyles of the young Italians at the time of the squadristi and futurism in the 1920s all indicated political affiliations.

The length of the hair and the shape and presence of beards and moustaches is a source of unending interest. Sometimes long hair has been a sign of servility, at others of nobility; Greek Orthodox priests wear beards, but on the whole the

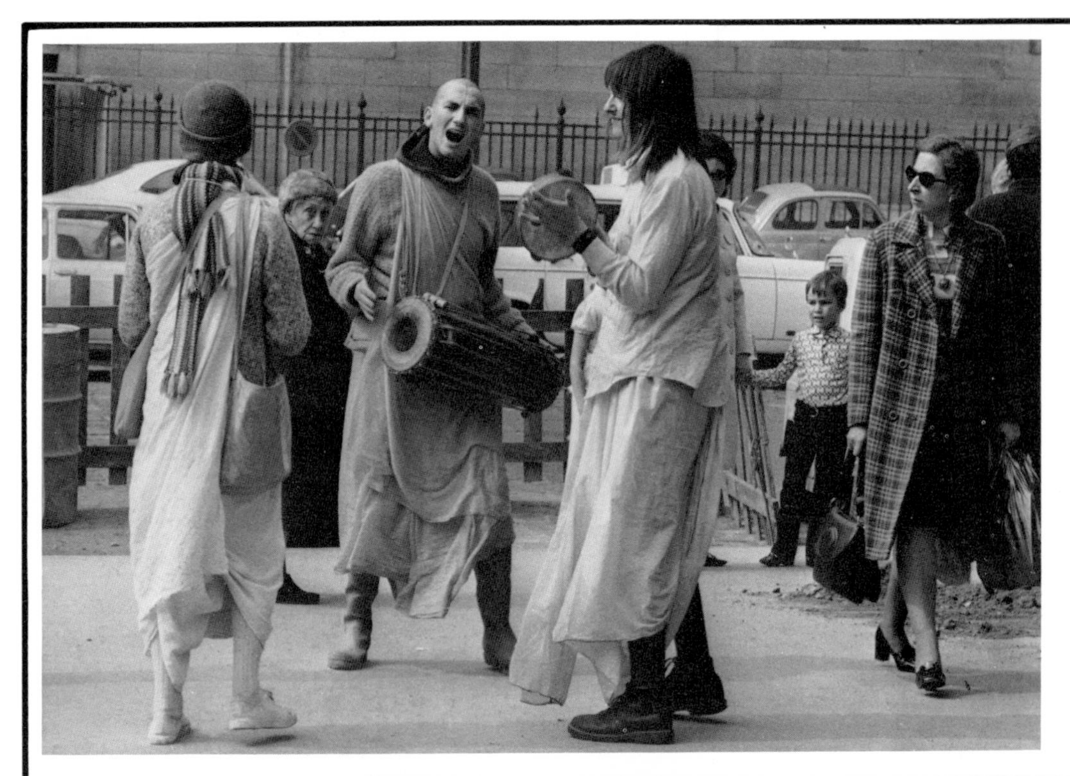

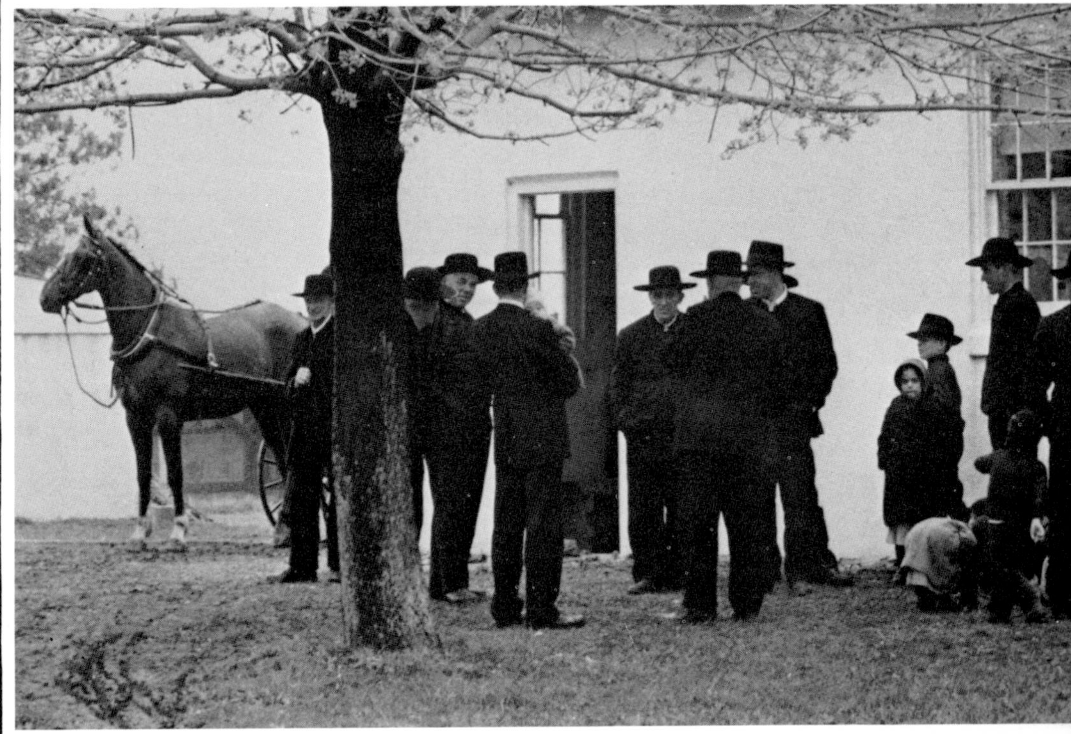

*Religious groups set themselves apart by their food and taboos, by special clothes, and by hairstyle and life style. Here the Conscience of Krishna sing in the streets of Paris.* below *The Amish of Pennsylvania, descendants of sixteenth-century Anabaptist immigrants from Europe, have kept their identity through their clothes, hairstyles and their way of life, which forgoes the embellishments of modern American civilization.*

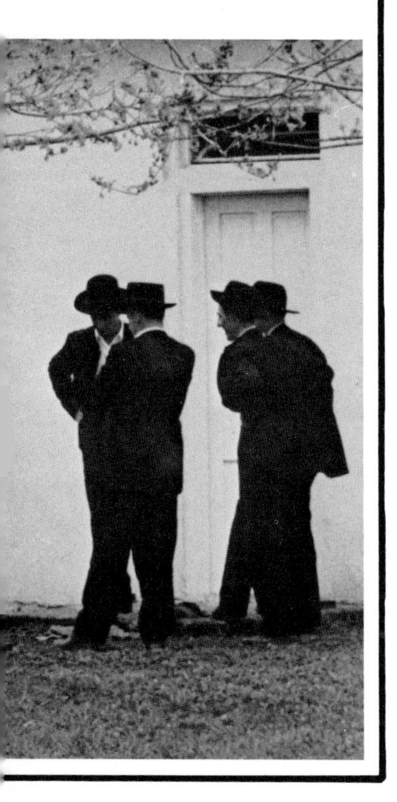

Christian Church does not favour them; in Ancient Egypt all but the nobility were clean shaven; in Ancient Greece all but the nobility were bearded; in Egypt, where beards were the unchallenged prerogative of rulers and the upper classes, they were worn in graded sizes according to rank, and even women wore artificial, ceremonial beards to mark their status and authority.

In modern Europe, hair has sometimes set groups apart. Certain shapes of wigs came to be associated with professions. In one of Henry Fielding's books a character says: 'I must have a physician's habit, for a physician can no more prescribe without a full wig than without a face.' Even military regiments had different styles of wig, distinguished either by shape or colour. The nicknames 'Buffs' (the Royal East Kent Regiment) and 'Blues' (the Royal Horse Guards) are derived from the colour of the powder dusted on the regimental wigs.

The United States Marine Corps physically and psychologically transforms a member of the wider society, a civilian, into a soldier. He is not tattooed or mutilated, but his image and general orientation which identify him with civilian life are stripped from him and his personal identity is suppressed as he is transformed into a marine. The marine's physical body is transformed; his head is shaved, his civilian wear is replaced by shapeless identical clothes, all vestiges of his former identity are removed. At first he is restricted to barracks and refused contact with the outside world. A degree of physical performance is demanded which few can meet; he is confused by complex demands; he is degraded by kicks on the rump, raps on the helmet, name calling, abuse and humiliating punishments. In the meantime, a shared bodily appearance, shared punishments and an *esprit de corps* with constant rewards for conformity weld the trainees together.

In the eighteenth century, the army insisted on a different kind of conformity: soldiers were obliged to wear pigtails and lovelocks. In the early nineteenth century they were required to wear moustaches, and young beardless youths were obliged to paint them on for uniformity's sake.

Even the religions use the body as an expression of belonging as well as belief. The Hara Krishna-ites set themselves apart from society by special body styles, dress and shaven heads. The Old-order Amish are an extreme example of the successful use of styles of dress and body ornament or lack of adornment in maintaining group isolation and a unique way of life. In 1525, when the Anabaptists came into being, the beard was commonly worn by men of all classes except Catholic priests. As early as 1568 the Anabaptists passed a resolution forbidding the trimming of the beard and hair. After the French Revolution, Napoleon's soldiers began wearing moustaches without beards, and in reaction to this practice and to set themselves apart the Mennonites (Anabaptists) and their stricter co-religionists, the Amish, shaved their upper lips. Both groups wanted nothing to do with the military and both groups have persistently opposed the moustache and war down to the present time. In America, this type of beard is known as the Täuferbart or Anabaptist beard. Amish men today wear their hair bobbed, cut below the ear or slightly above the earlobes. The hairstyle was common in eighteenth-century America, and the Amish have retained it as an index of belonging to the group. An Amish member is subject to the sanctions of the church if his hair is worn too short. Ornaments, make-up and tattoos are not allowed. Women's hair must be long and uncut, parted down the middle and combed down the sides. A girl's hair from infancy is braided, and from adolescence it is put up at the back. As far as body symbols are concerned, the Amish refuse to adopt signs of American civilization because they are not in sympathy with the 'worldly world'. Dress and hairstyle have become symbolic signs of an individual's attachment to the group: broad-brimmed hats for the men, black shawls for the women. The Amish also accentuate their distinctive culture by driving horses instead of cars and maintaining a semi-closed community through a spoken dialect known as Pennsylvanian Dutch.

*A hairstyle is a sign of religious persuasion. Rajasthani from the North-west Frontier.*

Other groups use similar methods to reinforce group bonding and withstand pressure from outside. Slang, hairstyles and clothes set modern gangs or groups apart. In England in the late 1940s the Teddy Boys sported a longish, greasy hairstyle with a straight neckline, along with side-whiskers and quiffs. the bootlace tie, thick crepe shoes and skin-tight trousers. Rockers wore leather jackets and faded jeans, while the Mods had a smoother look. The creation of a distinctive body-style enabled them to enjoy status and acquire a sense of identity. Their style also set them apart, so that other groups and all kinds of outsiders—the police, social workers—could use the stereotypes of body appearance to label them and link them with particular kinds of behaviour.

Painting, hairstyles and wigs have one great disadvantage—they are temporary. Therefore certain groups have always

*A Papuan celebrates his nose by incorporating a tusk nose plug in it.*

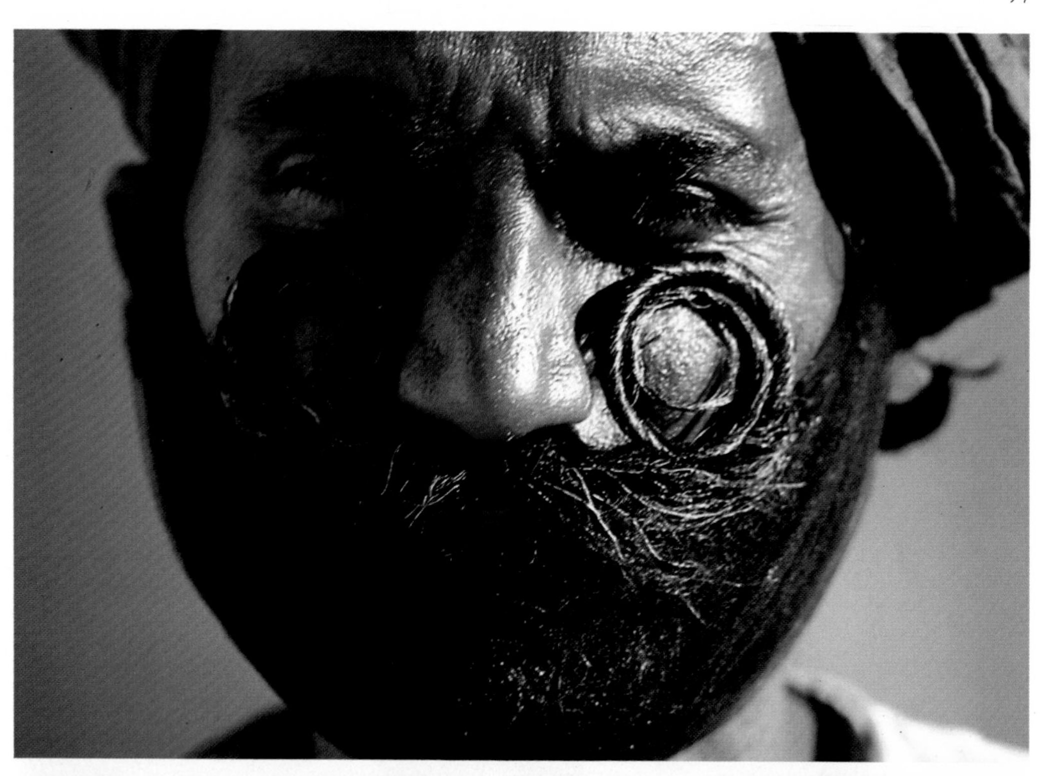

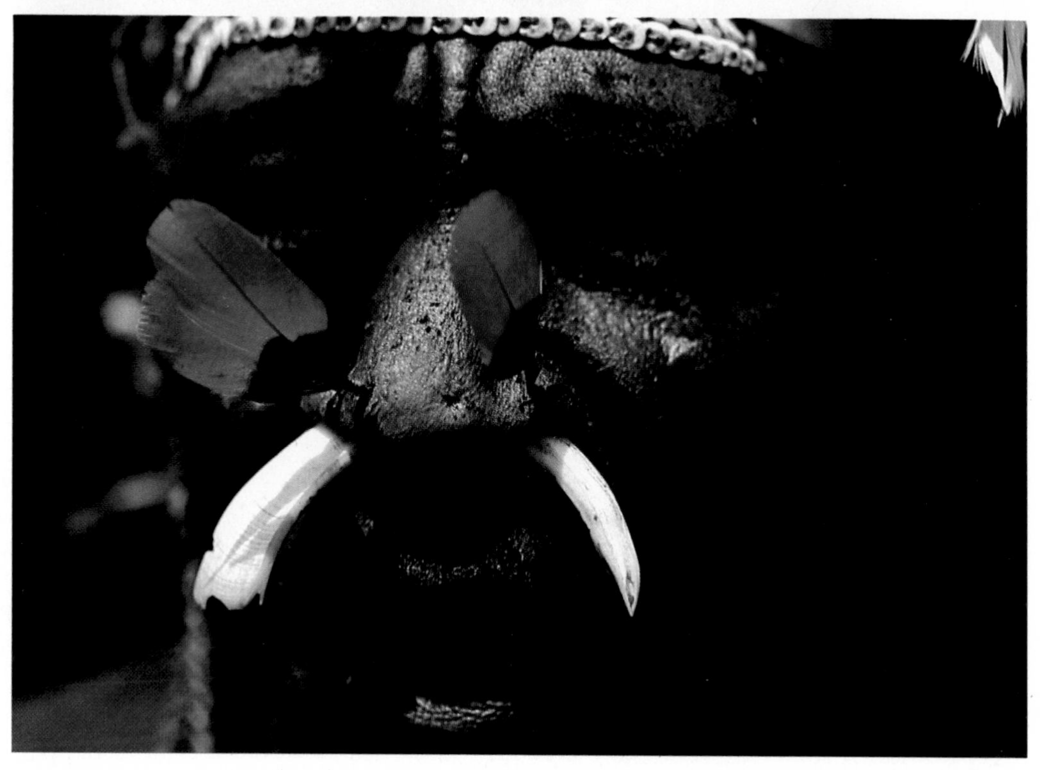

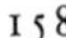

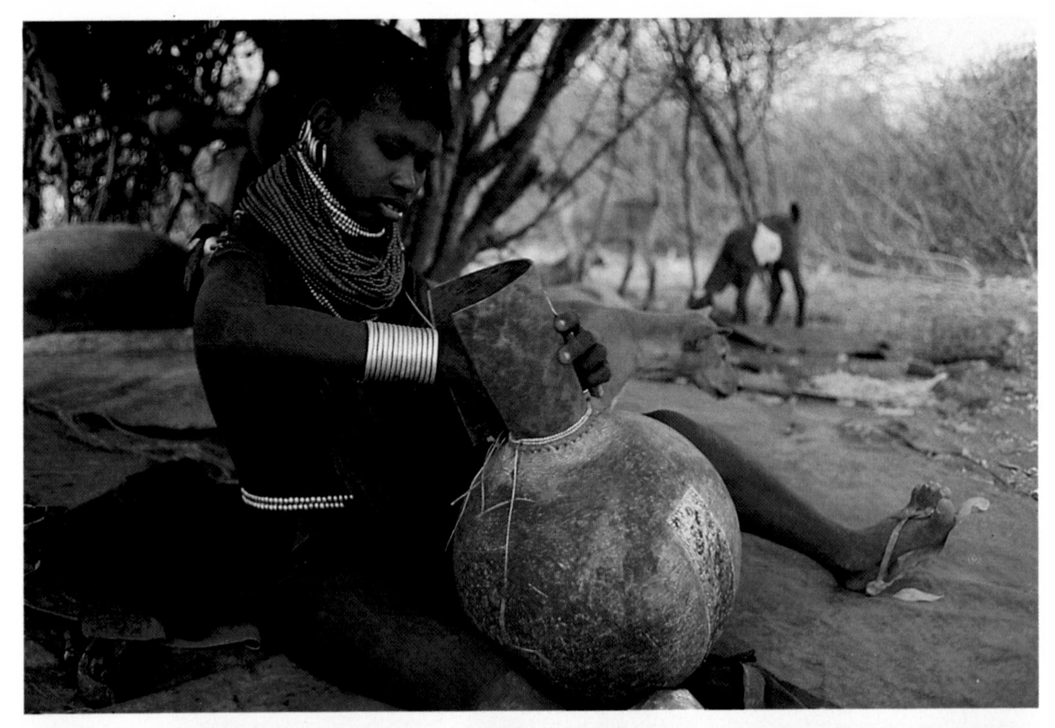

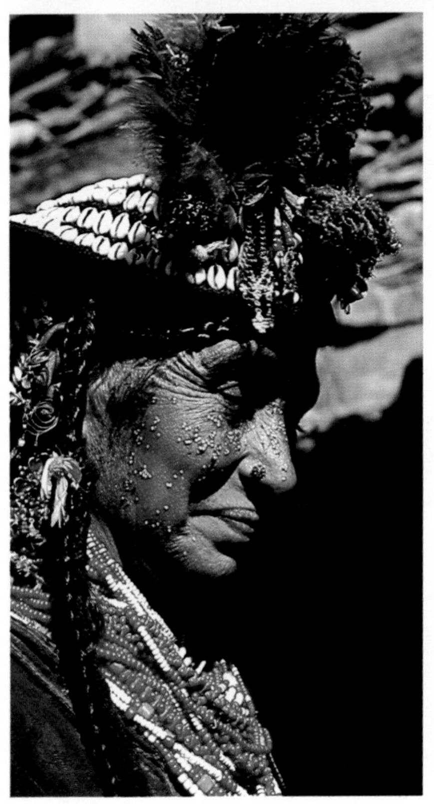

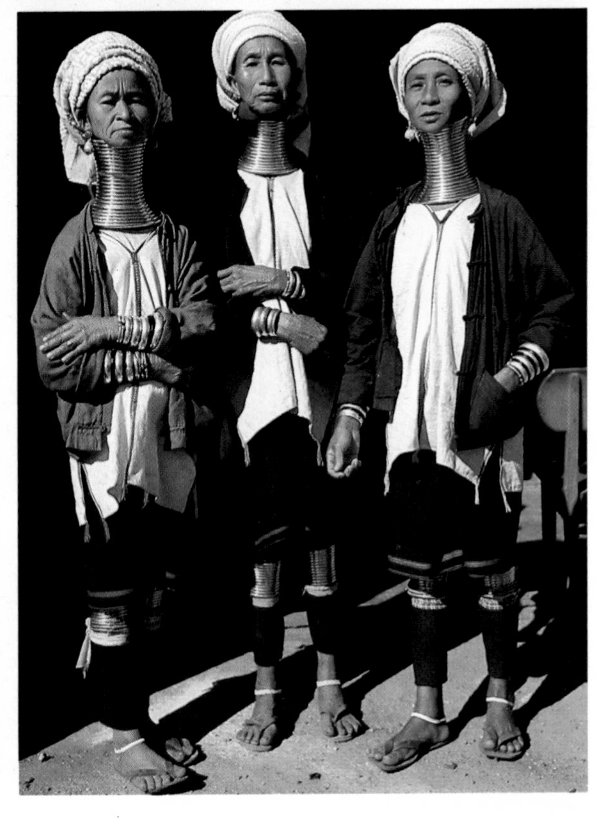

*Nomads (these are Turkana from Kenya), forced to travel light, often wear their wealth as ornamentation.*

wanted a more permanent symbol to express the nature of their membership. Members of European tradesmen's guilds were once tattooed with the appropriate symbol: the square, plumbline and trowel for masons; the crossed oven scoops for bakers; a lamp for miners. Today, certain social categories such as sailors, teenage gangs, Borstal boys and prison inmates seek to identify themselves as members of a group. In the early 1960s in England, a Liverpool gang adopted a bird motif on their hands; Hell's Angels are always tattooed; even among drug addicts special signs are commonly seen, including dots on the hands, arrows and syringes which point to the venous channels, or spiders and other dark insects tattooed over the tell-tall scars. Punk rock adolescents violently dye their hair, pierce their noses, cheeks and ears, and in other ways maltreat their skins, thereby, reputedly, sending out anti-authoritarian and political messages.

Generally, in our society, it has been people condemned to a permanently low status who have traditionally indulged in tattooing. It may seem a far cry from the elegant art of Maori *moko* or Japanese *irezumi* to the rough and ready tattooing of European prisons, but even here the social function of tattooing may be similar. As in *moko*, tattooing can reflect the rank and status of individuals, or as in *irezumi* the low status of certain social groups. Big-shots in French prisons had the most elaborate tattoos. 'Takes more than that for the guy to deserve a tattoo for big shots', says a character in Jean Genet's *Miracle of the Rose*. 'If he ever tattoos with anything but a flower, I'll attend to him myself.' Tattooing in these prisons celebrated rank and also celebrated sentiments of belonging.

> We had our bodies tattooed with adornments so that the flower and scroll would be set in a framework worthy of them. Some were cruelly branded with brutal signs that ate away their flesh like lovers' initials graven on aloe leaves. I would gaze with anguish at the men who were devoured by drawings as the crews of galleys were by salt, for the tattoos were the mark—stylized, ornate and flowery, as all marks become, whether they grow more intricate or less—of the wounds they would suffer later on, sometimes in the heart, sometimes on their flesh, whereas in days of old, on the galley, pirates had those frightful ornaments all over their body, so that life in society became impossible for them. Having willed that impossibility themselves, they suffered

far left *A Kalash-Kafiristani woman from Pakistan, elaborately made up and ornamented. Rice is included in her make-up.*
left *Padaung women from Burma wear neck rings, symbols of their status and of their submission to their husbands. The distortion caused to their necks parallels the distortion caused to Western women's torsos through tight lacing.*

less from the rigour of fate. They willed it, limited their universe in its space and comfort.

In fiction, Genet has explained more about the nature of European tattooing than the long tomes written by criminologists and sociologists on the phenomenon of body deformation since the nineteenth century.

Criminologists in the last century, such as Lacassagne and Lombroso, decided to their own satisfaction that to mutilate the skin by tattooing you had to be mad, bad or perverted; tattooing was the prerogative of the uneducated and criminal classes. Lombroso, after examining nearly 7,000 tattooed persons, including 3,000 criminals, stated that 'one of the most characteristic traits of primitive man . . . is the readiness with which he submits to this operation.' Tattooing was held to be an atavistic trait which had persisted among the lower classes.

Today, people are still worrying why certain groups maltreat their skin. In prison surveys in France it was found that ten per cent or so were tattooed on entering prison, but when the sentence was completed, the majority were marked. In British and American prisons the figures are over fifty per cent. One of the most important impulses behind tattooing seems to be a search for identity in a precarious situation. (There is also a magical element: sailors may use Christian symbols for protection—a cross tattooed on the back, for instance, magically alleviated the pain of flogging; in the United States, on the other hand, a pig tattooed on the left instep was an infallible charm against drowning.) Those in dangerous occupations, such as deep-sea fishermen, sailors, soldiers and criminals attempt to create a sense of identity by tattooing, just as the Maori *moko* impressed a personality on the face of its wearer.

Lombroso maintained that criminals tattooed themselves because they were born criminals and born tattooers. Yet we find that more often these deprived groups are actually branded with tattoos by the authorities. In Japan, those who were convicted of robbery were marked with a cross, and for each additional crime a similar tattoo was added, so that when brought for trial the criminal was marked with his previous convictions. Similarly, up to 1876 the British Army had special letters tattooed on the wrists of bad characters (B.C.) and deserters (D.). In Burma, criminals were tattooed with a circle in blue on the cheek and their name on the forehead. Throughout history, tattooing has been a convenient mode of branding

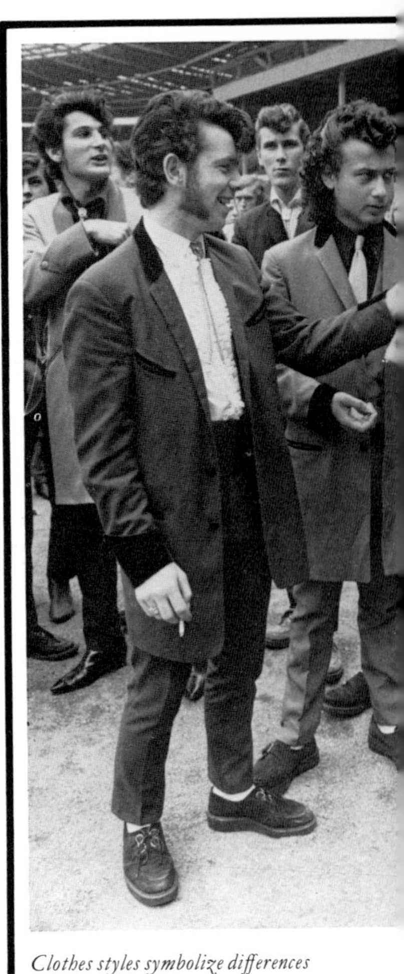

*Clothes styles symbolize differences between various youth groups in modern society. Teddy Boys* (above) *have dressed up for a Rock 'n' Roll revival show. In the case of the Punk Rock youth* (top right), *violently dyed hair and maltreated skin is an anti-establishment and anti-authoritarian message. Certain social groups—sailors and deep-sea fishermen, ex-convicts and Borstal boys—create a sense of identity by tattooing. In some cases, the separation of the group from normal society (in the case of these sailors* (right) *from land-lubbers) results in body marking as a symbol of defiance.*

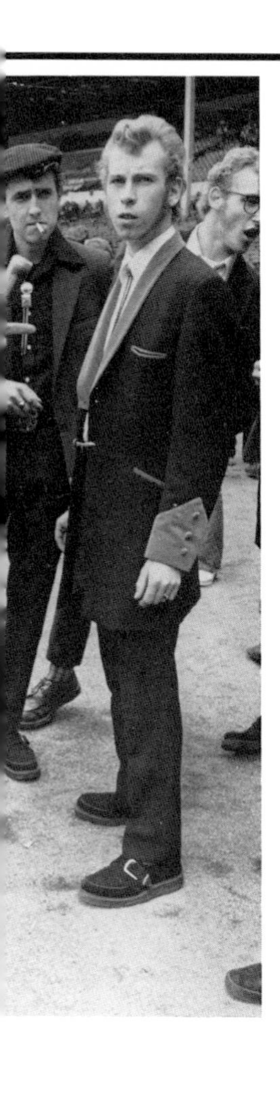

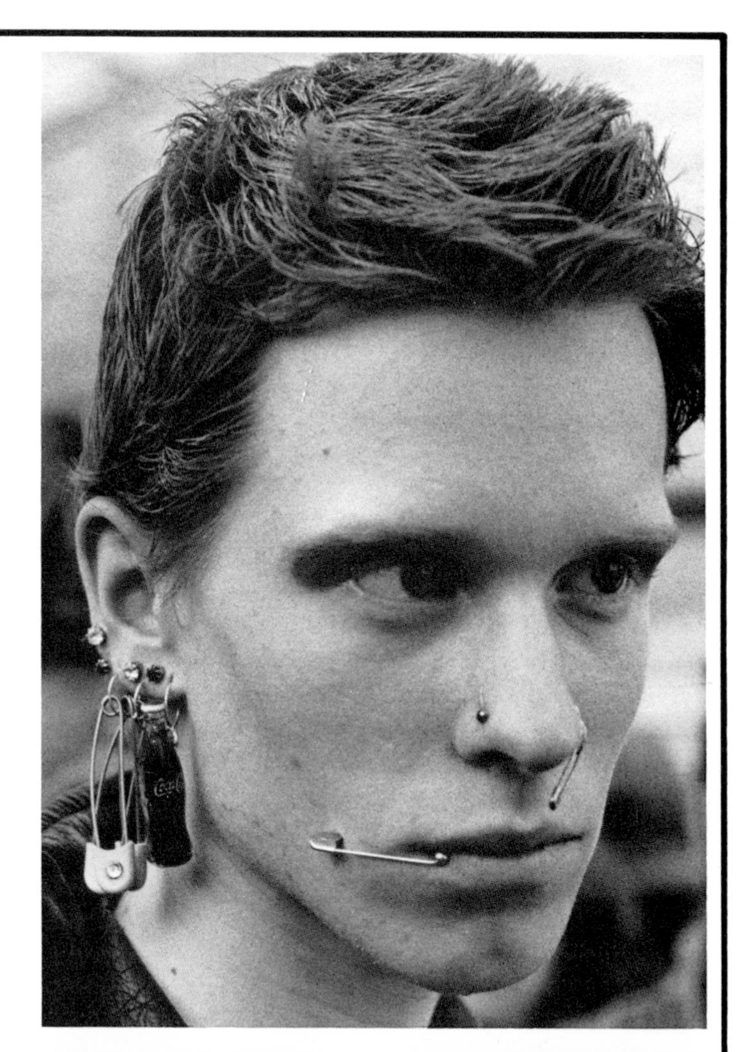

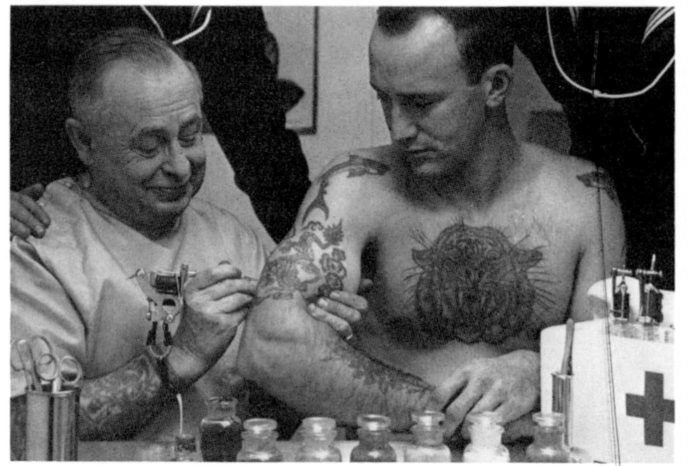

criminals and slaves.

In the West, tattooing is still common among ex-convicts, Borstal boys and girls and soldiers. It seems that the separation of a group from normal society results in body marking as a symbol of defiance. French prisoners write 'death to the police' or 'vengeance'. Formerly, solitary confinement was indicated by a lily on the shoulder, a year's imprisonment by wooden clogs; thieves had butterfly designs; gamblers dice. In British and American prisons, convicts tattoo such slogans as 'fuck the cops' or 'I'm a rebel'. It is natural enough for people outside the law to have tattoo marks and sentiments expressing their hatred of society or their disillusionment; moreover, a sense of diminished personality is often achieved or counteracted by attention to the body.

The use of tattooing among deprived groups depends very much on the fact of its permanence. There is absolutely nothing to be done to stop tattooing in modern prisons, and even among Borstal girls tattooing is compulsive. Girls puncture their skins with needles and rub ink into the wounds with ballpoint pens or use pigment from watercolour paints. The remarkable thing is that the great majority of the girls are repelled by the tattooing when they leave prison, and many are treated by plastic surgery or they remove the marks themselves with bleach and acid or alter them with razors and knives.

It is now clear that the desire for tattoos cannot be attributed to hereditary disturbed states of mind, the masculinity of female inmates or even boredom. The girls at a Borstal all express an obsession with life inside the institution, maintaining that tattoos make them feel good, give a permanent record of their friends, demonstrate their love and above all unite them all into a solidarity group.

Elsewhere, the members of a whole society, tribe or nationality may wear a mark, tattooed, painted or scarified, as a sign of belonging to the social group. In modern society, particularly in the United States, physical differences are almost an insult to the ideals of community conformity. The tattooing of gangs and groups is considered antisocial, since it symbolizes individual allegiances to ideals outside the ideals of mass democratic society. Tattooing and scarification on the skin of a drug addict, a Punk or an ex-convict are permanent reminders that these individuals have refused to conform, and authorities struggle ceaselessly to suppress the marks just as they struggle to suppress the anti-social groups.

Body decoration in the West today is therefore not expected to express symbols of social relations, ritual or mystical states, but to conform to a general American ideal. The modern beauty cult is closely linked with a contemporary passion for conformity.

*chapter ten*

# The Religious Body

*During the great Australian rituals, particularly the totemic food-increase rites, the men decorate themselves with sacred signs associated with the totemic ancestors. Once painted, the painter becomes the hero of the Dreaming, and enacts events of his mythical life.*

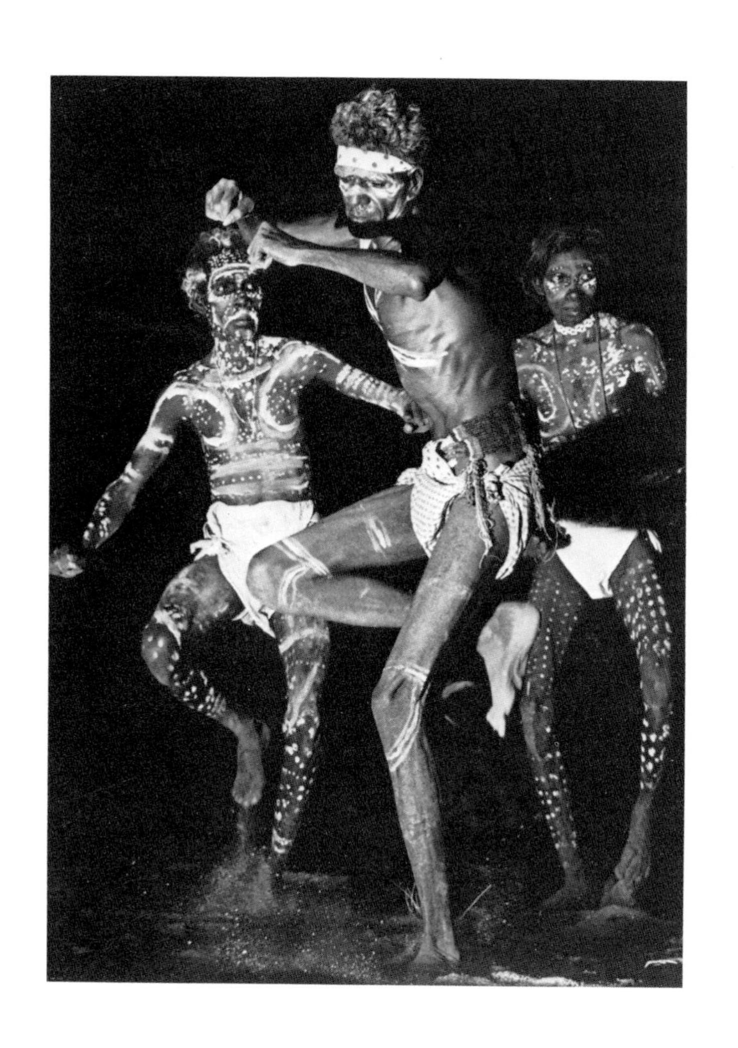

THE DECORATED BODY may become a shrine, a canvas imbued with religious significance and moral meaning. For us, for whom the physical body has always been a source of fears and sin, the flesh a weakness rather than a strength, it is difficult to comprehend the idea of a skin painted, tattooed or scarified in praise of a god. The body as a canvas for the spirit is no part of Christian iconography. Yet we find in Ancient Europe breasts and arms tattooed with the names and symbols of gods. In the Middle East, Islamic symbols are used as part of a decorative and curative art based on the body, and even in Christian Europe the tattooer haunted places of pilgrimage to imprint on the believer the signs of his devotion.

Among Hindus, the painted body (and even rules of hygiene) are closely connected with religious beliefs. Siva worshippers, for example, cover the forehead and various parts of the body with cowdung ashes or with ashes taken from the place where the dead are burnt; some smear the body from head to foot, others paint broad bars across the arms, chest and belly in memory of the long penance of Siva. The Nagas of East Assam think of the *tilaka* or caste mark on the forehead as a diminutive human shape and guard it from the infectious influence of strangers with an attached wormwood leaf, an effective disinfectant against the evil spirits. Generally in Hindu thought the *tilaka* is a sign of the seat of the soul and it is painted on the forehead as part of a general Hindu code. A bare forehead is a sign of mourning and fasting; but the presence of the *tilaka* also indicates that the daily ritual ablutions have been performed; before these ablutions, with the forehead bare, the person is in a state of impurity.

While examining body art, we have had glimpses of ritual and religious meaning, even if these beliefs were once patronizingly styled 'magic' and 'supernaturalism'. It is only since thorough anthropological researches began after the turn of the century that we have been able to try to piece together the role of the body arts in the cosmological beliefs of the Polynesians, Australians and Amerindians. In many cases it was too late.

One example which still remains is the common South American habit of smearing the head and hair with red paint. Among the Bororo of the Rio Xingu in Brazil, the head and hair must be painted red as one of the necessary precautions taken after death and for the proper celebration of the funeral feast. S. R. Karsten, who has written a copious book on South American body painting (hoping to reveal the magical nature of primitive paint), writes:

> When such hair-painting is resorted to . . . there are sufficient reasons for assuming that it is meant to serve, not any ornamental, but purely practical and magical purposes: to protect the hair, which being the seat of the soul, is one of the most critical parts of the body, against the ghost of the dead, or against other evil spirits which are then especially feared.

Karsten notes the supernatural nature of Bororo body painting, but in his association of primitive decorative practices with magic and supernatural protection we are merely left with a picture of simple savages daubing their heads through some childish superstition. A more recent account links social fact, symbol and rite, so that the role of painting the body red becomes a reasonable, culturally satisfying business.

The Yanomamo Indians of southern Venezuela and the neighbouring portions of northern Brazil are tonsured and have pudding-basin haircuts. At about the age of three, a child is formally given a name and the crown of his head is shaven. At this point he is considered to have acquired his individual human soul and his own personality. The Yanomamo describe this tonsure as a graphic representation of the moon's disc—the moon, and the moon's master the Lord of the World, being their most important deity. Throughout his or her life, the tonsure plays an important part in the social expression and ritual of each Yanomamo, and it is carefully tended, usually by the women, who cut and shave the heads of their kin every four weeks or so. At feasts and rites and prior to war expeditions, the tonsure is covered with a red plant dye. At the same time, it is tended, oiled and cleaned to keep the head free from lice. The Yanomamo are an aggressive people and their ferocity is often stimulated by drugs, particularly before competitive feasts, chest-pounding contests, duelling and organized raiding parties. During club fights, pieces of wood over two metres long are aimed at the opponent's head, so that the tops of most men's heads are covered with proud scars kept cleanly shaved for display. It is also on the tonsured head, and only there, that a husband may hit his wife.

What is the significance of the red-painted, battle-scarred Yanomamo tonsure? The anthropologist, asking a few more questions than the traveller interested only in tales of magic and violence, discovers that Pore, the Yanomamo 'man in the moon', Lord of the World, is conceived of as an old man with a long white beard and the same red-dyed tonsure which is prescriptive for all Yanomamo. It is the red-painted head which forms a kind of ground structure for the cosmological beliefs associated with Pore and the moon. The tonsure is envisaged as the mirror image of the moon, and the Yanomamo imagine the moon as a disc covered with lakes of blood, while on this disc Pore, the great spirit being, walks like men walk on Earth, but upside down. So the head of the Yanomamo, facing the moon, is a symbol of the terrestrial world, while the tonsure itself is a representation of the moon and its lakes of blood.

*A shaven head may be a mystical sign. Cayapo Indians from South America are depicted here. Among some Indian peoples a tonsure was a graphic representation of the moon's disc.*

When a Yanomamo dies, the corpse is cured and the soul escapes up to the moon in smoke, later returning beneficently to the Earth as drops of blood, which, hitting the clouds, fall as rain. This blood-rain is associated with a tree that grows in the middle of the moon, and it is this tree, known as the Rain Tree, which is the life symbol of the Yanomamo. They liken their own bodies to this tree: the head and specially the tonsure on the crown is the top of the tree and the hair its leaves; the arms are the branches and the skeleton, where the soul lives, its trunk. The human skin is the bark, while the body itself is the external shell. For the Yanomamo, the important substance is the soul stuff found in the bones; at rebirth this soul-substance always goes to a person of the opposite sex. The soul-substance of the bones, set in the body of blood, is likened to the lakes of blood on the moon; and the hairstyle and red paint are the outward signs of the real nature of the Yanomamo as moon-dwellers. When they dance in honour of their ancestors they wear fluffy feathers and kapok in their hair, symbols of clouds and peace, clouds representing important links between Earth and the moon. Women are tattooed on their upper lip with the sickle moon at first menstruation, and in some ways, because they have 'more blood' than men, they are considered closer to the moon.

Now, although I do not pretend that such a brief description of Yanomamo beliefs about the head, the body and the moon can bring us anywhere near a complete understanding of their religion, we have at least a hint of its complexity, a hint of the interrelationship of social life, body art and cosmology.

Another people who are inveterate and lavish body painters are the Australians, as we have seen. During the great ceremonies and rituals, particularly the *intichuma* or food-increase rites, the men decorate themselves with sacred signs asso-

*Two Bathurst Islanders taking part in the Purukupali (Moon Myth) dance. In mythical times, Tapana, the moon, stole Waiei, the wife of Purukupali, while the latter was out hunting. Without his parents, their baby son Djinani died, and Tapana undertook to bring the boy back to life within three days. Purukupali refused and said that everyone must now die. There was a fight, and Tapana lost, returning to the sky where his wounds are still visible on the moon's surface. Purukupali, grief-stricken, drowned himself; Waiei turned into a curlew and her sad cries are heard as she searches for her child. The illustration shows Purukupali fighting Tapana.*

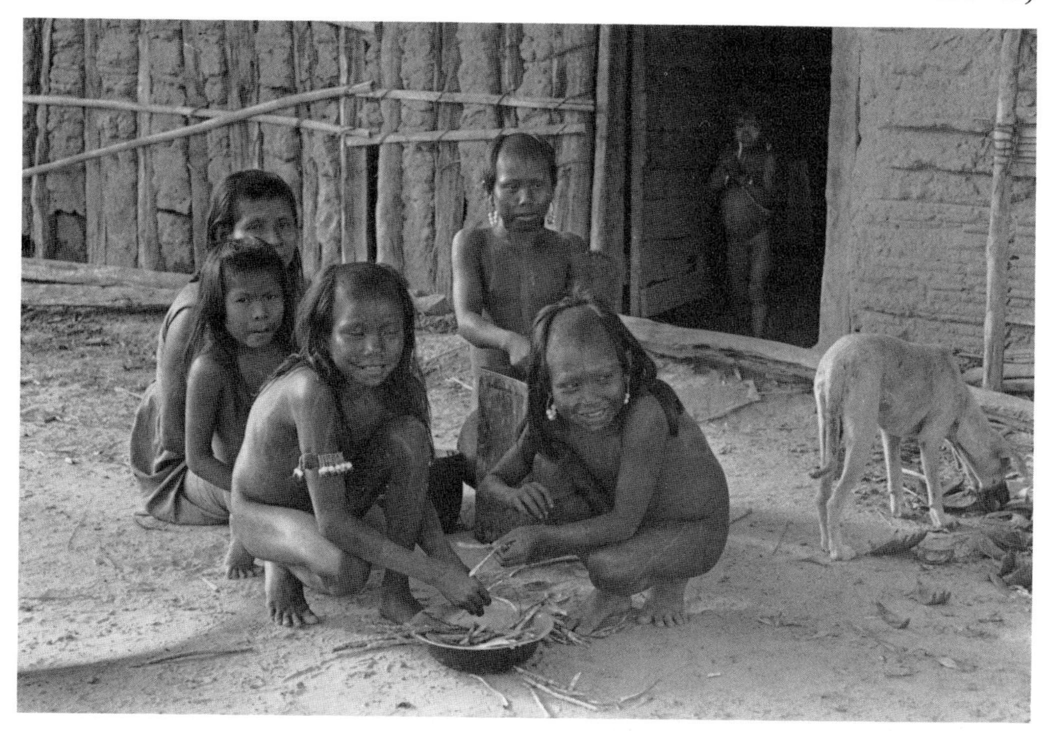

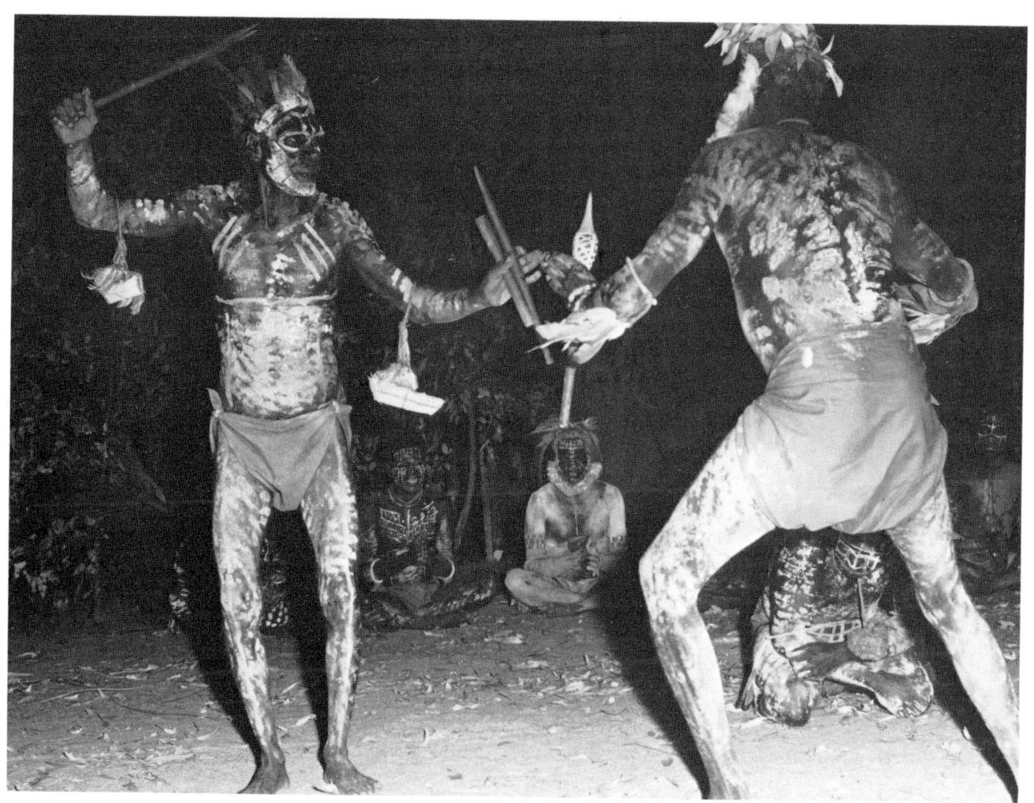

ciated with the totemic ancestors, those taking part being painted with patterns that belong to their ceremonial groups or clans. During the long process of painting the body and adding the down with blood-fixative, a cycle of songs describing the life and deeds of the culture heroes is sung. Once the painting is complete, the dancer becomes the hero, the hero of the dreaming, and enacts events of his mythical life. The ordinary mortal, by washing and anointing the body, being smeared with red ochre and designs outlined in clay, completed with down stuck on with blood, becomes a god. As soon as the scene is over, the painting is obliterated with red ochre. It has served its purpose, symbolizing a particular hero and a particular event, and as the decoration is wiped off, the totemic spirit disappears.

*Western cosmetics celebrate sexuality and vanity. In other parts of the world body art has religious and ritual meaning. The meaning of the Australian totemic dances has for the most part been lost, early observers merely referring to their 'magical corroborees'.*

In the Australian ceremonial dances, the mythical being emerges from the sacred totemic sites in the form of a painted dancer. Almost every part of the body is used for these basically religious transformations. The designs begin on the face and continue to the loins, spreading over and across the shoulders to the back, then down the thighs to just above the knees. The men also wear head-bands, nose bones and bunches of feathers. Even the didgeridoos and the boomerangs are decorated, and the *churinga*, symbolic objects of wood and stone, are painted with the sacred patterns associated with the totems.

Most Australian body painting was observed in the nineteenth century and suffers, like that of the South Americans, from prejudiced and subjective explanations and over-attention to technique and patterns. Australian designs must be studied in context, since the signs themselves are somewhat remotely related to the objects they are meant to represent. Only informed clan elders can explain the meaning; but for them every line, every dot, every segment of colour is an element in the general symbolic pattern which represents the myth and history of the totemic group.

Fortunately, the designs of one Australian people, the Walbiri, have been studied on the spot, in detail and in context, by the American anthropologist Nancy Munn. She has analysed the signs, the ceremonies and the accompanying songs as part of a process which links the Australian to his gods and individuals to each other in a social setting. Suitably enough, she worked mainly among women, though their designs are restricted to the ceremonies they may attend and to signs and symbols appropriate to women. There are in fact

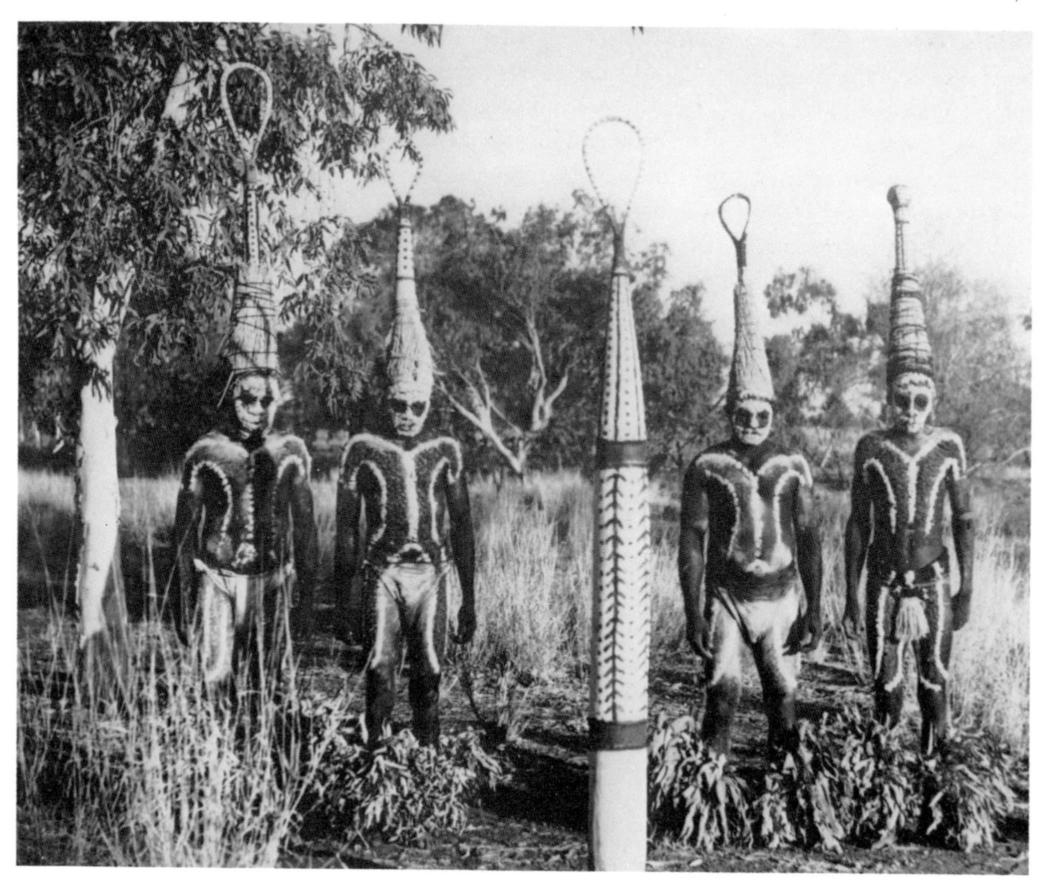

two kinds of women's painting: one is performed along with men's ceremonies, especially the circumcision rites; the other is performed independently, and its main purpose is to attract lovers. The signs reflect women's interest in sexuality and procreation, health and the growth of children, but they are also believed to promote the growth of plants and other foods specially associated with women.

Among these Walbiri women, designs are painted on the body with red ochre, charcoal and a white paste made from friable stone. Decorations are applied with a small string-bound stick or with the fingers to the breast and across the shoulders to the upper arms, stomach and thighs. Individual women may dream their designs and regard them consequently as their personal property, sharing them with relatives and co-wives. Several species of ancestors (or totems) are emphasized in the paintings: rain, two forms of berry, the honey ant, the opossum (phalanger) and charcoal fire. These are the spirits of food collected by women, while rain has strong feminine associations and the charcoal fire ancestors were female. The signs representing the totems follow the shape of the body. Thus, lizard patterns are painted on movable parts such as legs and arms. Some designs on the breasts and shoulders are distorted to accommodate the curve of the breasts, so that the honey ant becomes elongated or curved, while on the arm it is a more usual representational shape.

Women's paintings, like the tattooing and scarification of women which we have already discussed, are connected with woman's biological role. A girl is painted at birth, at first menstruation and before going to her husband for the first time, when her breasts are decorated to make them grow and make the milk come.

Men's ritual designs are quite another matter. Women are excluded from their execution and do not usually see them. They are associated with ceremonial regalia: headdresses, ground paintings, *churinga* boards (painted in ochres or incised and rubbed with ochre), as well as bullroarers and shields. The designs painted on the ceremonial objects are also painted on the body with red and yellow ochres, white and black paints, all on a grease base. For increase ceremonies, red ochre and white fluff are used, which create a kind of overall mask by obscuring the face and torso in a covering of designs. The increase ceremonies take place at the same time as the initiation rites, when young men are circumcised; song cycles are sung and ancestral events of the dreaming are dramatized as part of the general fertility ceremony.

Nancy Munn shows that the functions of the designs are bound up with ideas of procreative sexuality and the generative potency of the ancestors. They are graphic condensations of vital fertility symbols, usually found in dreams. The designs attain their potency through the association of the symbols of sexuality and fertility and the body on which they are painted. Designs and songs intoned during the ceremony are closely related: the painted designs immediately bring to mind the songs which are symbols of the designs, and vice versa.

Men's designs are homogeneous in general effect, with an infinite variety of small detail, a fact which correlates with an earlier remark about painting in Arnhem Land, where the basic pattern is a clan pattern and details are individual additions. Elements in the patterns include camp-sites, paths, the lightning-snake-smoke syndrome, human beings, caves, the rainbow, and spears, and each ancestor is associated with the distinctive features of a totemic species. There may be linked species occurring together in a design. Wallaby and dingo footprints may appear with snake tracks because they are said, in myth, to have crossed the ancestral track in ancient times. The ancestral beings are being made visible in body painting through abstract signs. They are symbols which have implications for human reproduction as well as the reproduction of totemic species, many of which are related to food supplies. At increase ceremonies, groups are ritually producing food for other groups, since to eat one's own totemic species is usually taboo. Again we see the emphasis on mutual aid between clans which we found expressed in the 'trading' of ceremonial clan designs among Arnhem Land Australians.

During the increase ceremonies, the dancers, with their ceremonial paraphernalia and body painting, reconstruct the ancestor, and as part of this process, a process involving painting, singing and dancing, they help the continuation of essential food in the country as a whole. In effect, if the dancers belong to the red kangaroo clan, they are embodying the totemic kangaroo ancestor, as well as the kangaroo family. During the ceremonies, the hero, the cultural ancestor, the totem, is created by his descendants in his procreative capacity, and by dancing he—or his descendants—maintains the continuity of the species and the land.

Australian designs reflect this preoccupation. The dancer's face and torso are covered with decorations, his physical skin overlaid with forms and designs reflecting the identity of the ancestor. Women's designs are focused on the personal, family aspects of life; men's are linked to the wider social structure, based on descent, and to the clan in its ritual and ceremonial role.

While the body as a shrine or canvas demonstrating a people's ties with their gods or their ancestors can be clearly seen as a religious body, the natural developments of the human body, from birth to death, can also be examined in the light of a religious—binding—acknowledgement of Nature as she affects the human body, and this we shall examine in the next chapter.

*chapter eleven*

# Passage Rites

*In small communities the decorated body has a ritual significance and distinguishes boys from girls, children from adolescents, adolescents from adults. This Tchikrin boy from Brazil has a tonsured head as an indication of his status as a 'little one'.*

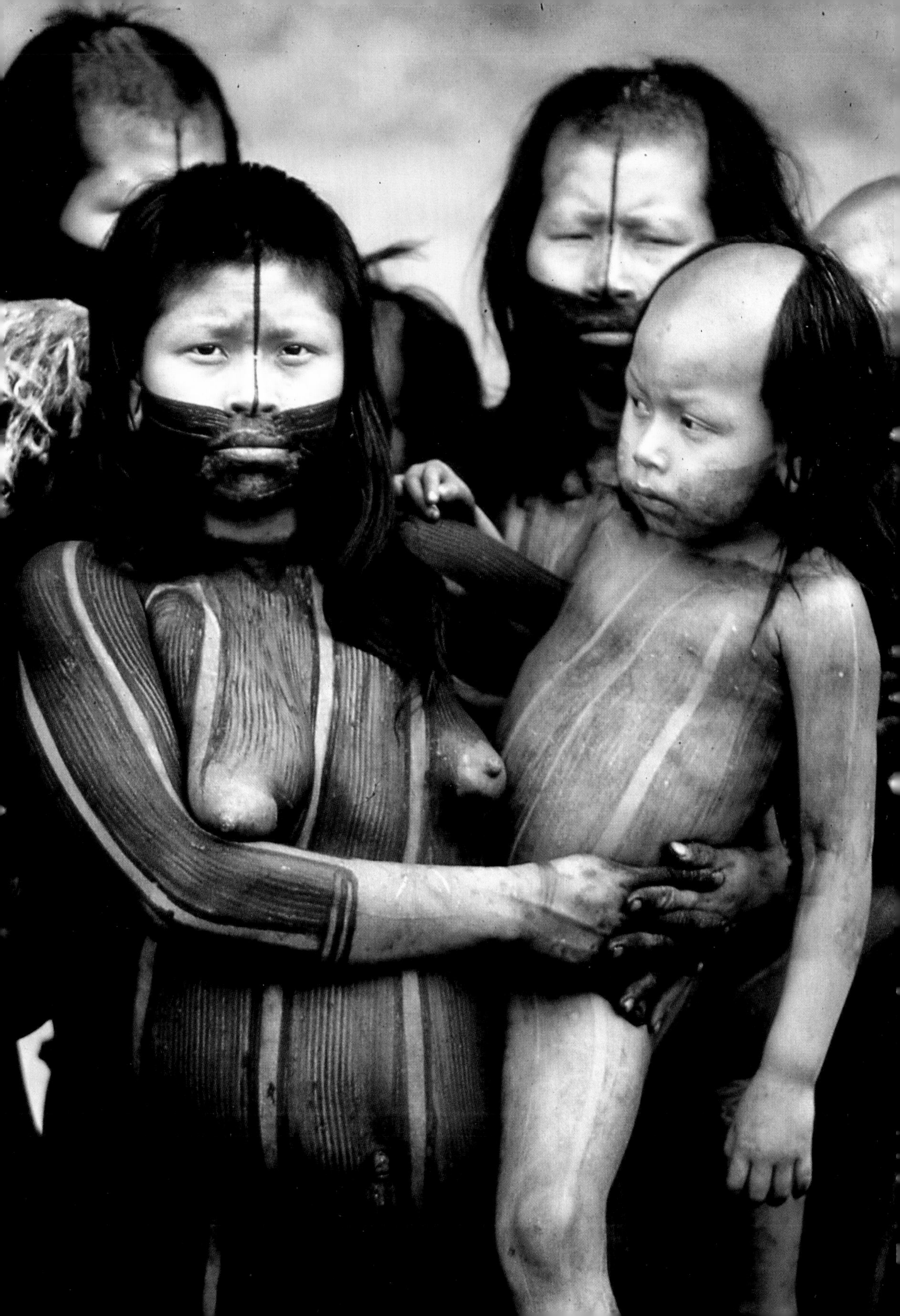

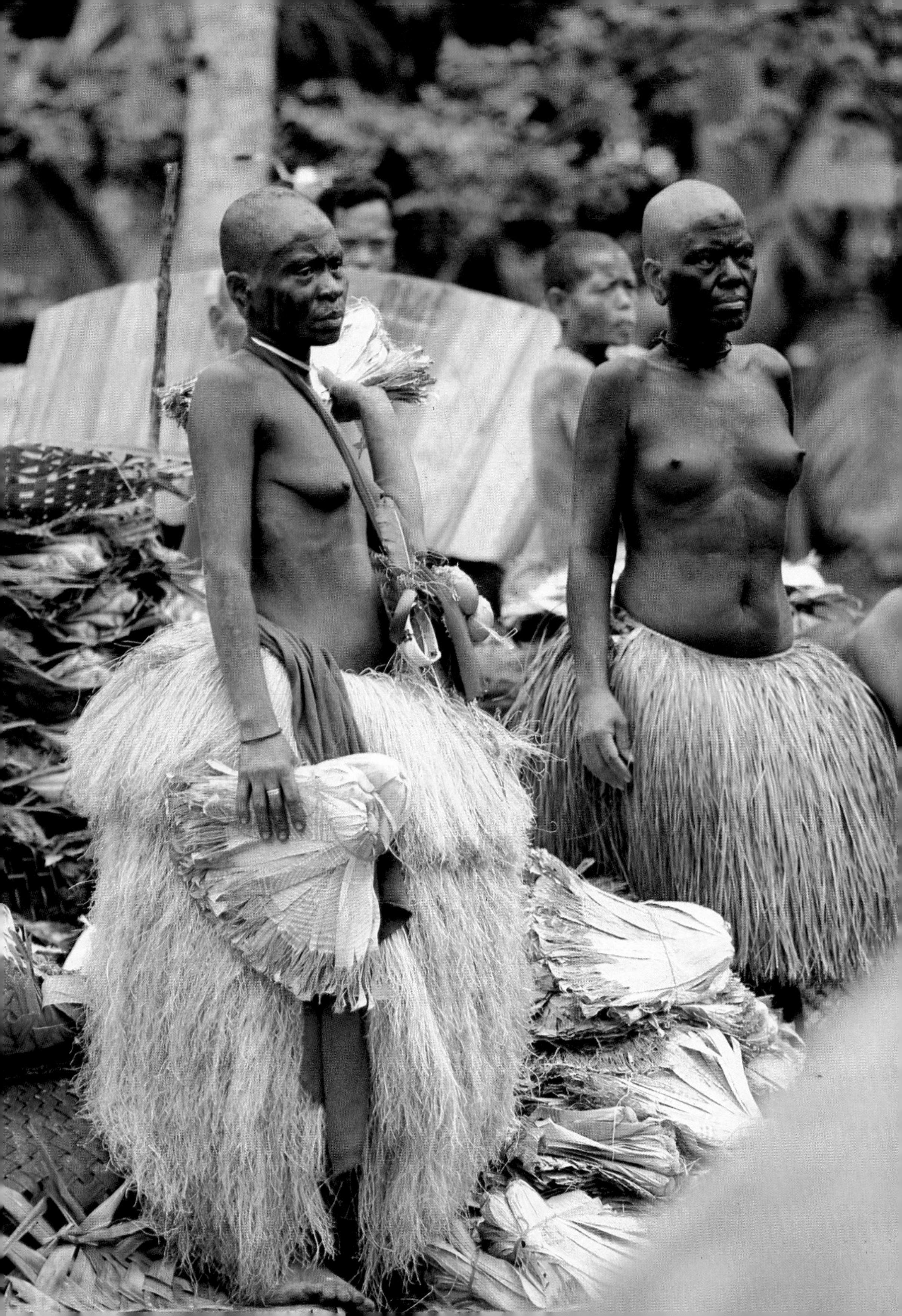

*Widows once wore 'weeds' and black veils in the West. In the Trobriands, women are painted and their heads shaved as a public sign of their widowhead.*

THERE ARE CERTAIN occasions, both public and private, when cosmetics or some form of body decoration are peculiarly appropriate. Some people paint before embarking on a journey or at particular times of the year, rather in the same way as we may celebrate Christmas Day or Thanksgiving Day with special foods.

Among the Karaya of eastern Brazil, it is the custom that on the arrival of guests in a village, both they and the hosts should be painted and adorned. When the guests arrive, the inhabitants of a whole village paint their faces with patterns of red and black, and the guests also decorate themselves before entering the village. Among other Orinoco peoples, the whole body is painted red for a visit, and on their arrival their paint, which has become messed by the journey, is renewed by the hosts. Guests of the Mbaya-Guaicuru used to don all their ornaments, including swords and lances, clothes and beads, when visiting. They stopped outside the village and on the following morning, all painted red, they entered the village, where the first greeting was a formal combat with fists.

A visit to another village, a journey, is a critical moment, and painting oneself serves to commemorate it.

During an individual's lifetime there are also critical moments when the body is marked as a sign of transition from one state to another. At birth, puberty, marriage and parenthood the body may be marked, either temporarily with paints or permanently with tattoos or scars. In *The Golden Bough*, for example, Frazer lists, besides the Jews of the Old Testament, over fifty examples in which some form of decoration or self-mutilation is practised at mourning; in almost every case we find that the cutting off of hair is accompanied by the wounding of the body.

Where people live in small communities, the decorated body has a much greater significance at ceremonies surrounding these important rites, although it may be true, as some writers have suggested, that our own cosmetic arts are employed at naturally critical periods. There are two particular moments in our lifetime in the West when we begin to worry about the appearance of our body and concern ourselves with grooming it: one is at puberty, when the adolescent starts to fear that he or she is not attractive; and the other at the 'change of life', when men and women begin to panic because they think their looks are fading, and attempt to forestall their inevitable physical decay with cosmetic aids.

In most societies, decoration plays an important part in

rites associated with these passages. Occasionally new hairstyles may be assumed: in West Africa, styles may distinguish little girls, nubile girls, a young bride, a mother, a widow, or even a woman who has lost her first child. Since passage rites change the personality of the individual, it is considered appropriate that the natural body should be transformed by decoration as a sign that it has changed from one status to the next. Again in West Africa, boys at puberty usually receive their first scarification. Among the Kabre of Togo they receive another set a few years later, when the head is shaved in public; and at the age of twenty or thereabouts, when they are considered to have reached adult male status, they acquire the final scars that make them full adult members of their group.

The birth of children to women is an important event, often marked by tattooing, painting or a new hairstyle. South American Indian fathers sometimes bleed themselves in the couvade (when they, instead of their wives, lie in child-bed in recognition of their new status of parenthood). Priests and chiefs may be marked during their rites of initiation and, finally, at death itself, the corpse may be marked or painted.

In our society the corpse is decorated for ostensibly aesthetic reasons—a touch of make-up, a little formaldehyde to plump out death's hollows. In other societies, the body is painted for frankly religious reasons. Sometimes the corpse is given a mark which acts as its passport to the next world. Among the Sioux Indians, elaborate precautions are taken for a dead man's safe and comfortable journey to the afterlife. The ghost-warrior mounts his ghostly steed and sets forth on his journey to the 'world of many lodges', with the confident feeling that he will arrive safely as long as he has the correct tattoo on his forehead, his wrist and the point of his chin. If the 'Old Woman' who examines ghosts finds no tattoo marks, he and his horse are pushed from a cliff or cloud and fall into a purgatory where they become homeless, aimless warriors. Even in Neanderthal burials, the importance of body art both before and after death is proved by the pots of red ochre placed near corpses as if they were provided with a supply of colour for the afterlife.

In South America, we have seen how the anthropologist studying the Suya stressed the symbolic role of ear-piercing and mouth-embellishment and their association with 'knowledge', 'obedience' and 'aggression'. Victor Turner, on the other hand, when describing the Tchikrin has shown how their body art marks the social progress of both sexes from

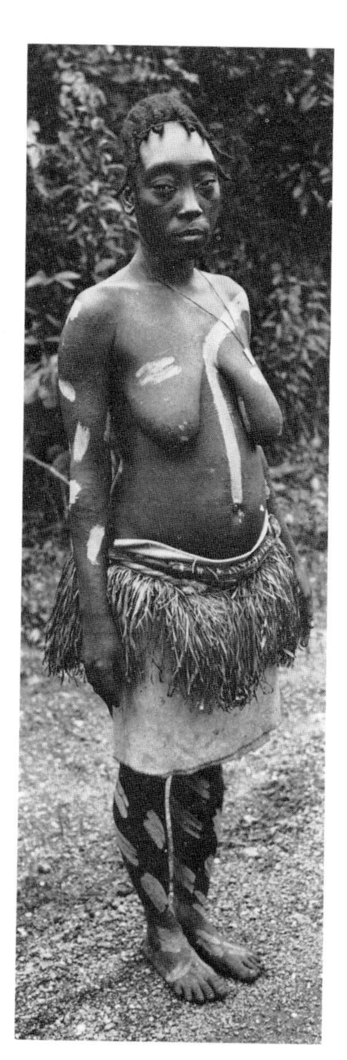

*A common sign of mourning throughout the world is the daubing of paint or clay or mud on the bodies of widows and children, as with this Mangbetu woman of Central Africa.*

birth to old age. The Tchikrin live in circular villages, with the huts disposed around a large central space. In these huts lives the typical extended Tchikrin family. Women are born here and stay put all their lives; boys move out at about the age of eight and go to live in the men's houses which are situated in the centre of the circular space. It is only after the consummation of their marriage by fathering a child that young men are allowed to move into their wives' houses. It is this progression from status to status which classifies a man into groups, or age grades, each with a distinctive style of body painting and ornamentation.

Boys and girls are elaborately decorated as babies. A few days after birth, the ear-lobes (and for a boy his lower lip as well) are pierced by the father. Cigar-shaped ear-plugs of reddened wood are inserted in the ears and replaced from time to time with larger ones until the holes in the lobes become very big. A string of beads is inserted in the boy's lower lip. The baby's body is kept painted by the mother, grandmother and other kinswomen, using a kind of stylus made from the centre rib of a leaf, and drawing complex linear patterns over the entire body. With their large wooden ear-plugs, their painted bodies, their plucked eyebrows and eyelashes, they are decorated as 'little ones'. As they grow up, every status change is marked by a change in body ornament or hairstyle. At weaning, when they walk and talk and when they are old enough to go to the men's houses, their bodies are ritually marked.

At the age of eight, when the boy is about to leave his family to live with an adopted, 'surrogate' father in the men's houses, he is stripped of his baby ornaments and his hair is cut. He is no longer painted by his mother in the style of infants, but in broad areas or bands of black and red, applied not with the midrib of a leaf but directly by hand. On moving, he is painted solid black, a colour ideally suited as a sign that he has been cut off from the world of the domestic family and has entered the world of men. The black paint of the Tchikrin boy marks the end of childhood and he now enters the new grade of older boys known as the 'painted ones'.

At puberty, there is another ceremony, associated with the acquisition of a penis sheath. At the same time the boy's lip ornaments are changed to the type of plugs worn by adult men and his hair is cut in the style of grown men and women. As among the Suya, the penis sheath is a symbolic expression of social control, and it and the new hairstyle publicly express the society's recognition of the growing boy's sexuality and his integration into the social structure, just as the progressive tattooing of a Motu girl's body symbolizes her status change from girl, to nubile woman, to married woman.

After the initiation at puberty, the boy is betrothed and has a right to mature sex. He is now a 'bachelor youth'; he marries when his betrothed is pregnant, and after founding a family he graduates to the grade of 'fathers' and joins the men's societies. These changes are again reflected in the final changes of the Tchikrin body. The boy's small lip plug is replaced by a larger, saucer-like plate, as much as four inches wide. There is an alternative form, made of a long cylindrical rock crystal or piece of wood.

A Tchikrin woman's progress is less complex, but when she becomes a potential sexual partner, mother and then wife, each new status is marked. In the puberty ceremonies, adoptive mothers paint the girls' thighs, breasts and upper arms in broad, black stripes. Now known as the 'black-thighed ones' they can consummate their courtships. When a woman has her third child, she is considered a socially mature adult, and she wears her hair long.

Body painting and scarification celebrate the passage rites of Australians from birth, when the newly born babies (and their mothers) are painted white, a decoration usually continued during the long suckling period. From that point on, the body is used as a veritable religious icon, temporary and permanent decoration marking status changes, which are normally accompanied by important religious ceremonies.

The gradual process of growing up is punctuated by the commas, semi-colons and full stops of ritual. A gentle mutilation—the cutting of a lock of hair—may mark a boy's first speared goanna (lizard). As new social status is achieved, teeth, skin, hair and body extremities are excised, patterned, altered, painted or scarified to proclaim the Australian's passage through life. For example, at menarche, the Australian girl is ritually 'made' into a woman through ceremonies accompanied by body decoration and special hairstyles. The girl retires to a secluded part of the camp with female relatives, who teach her the taboos associated with menstruation, and details of the group's moral and religious code. After a period of seclusion, she is bathed and makes a public entry into the main camp, accompanied by other women singing ceremonial songs. She is richly decorated, and acclaimed by

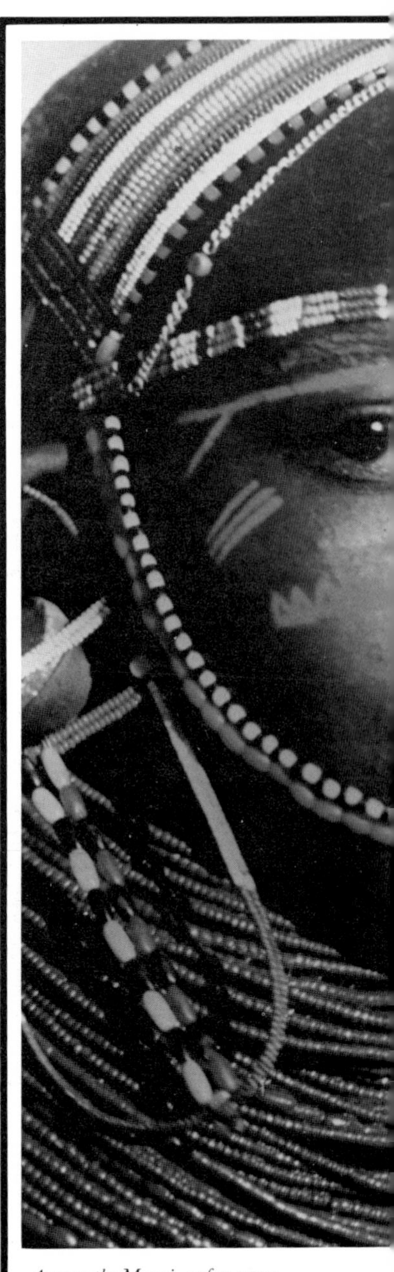

*Among the Masai, as for many African peoples, ceremonies confirm an individual's adulthood and their readiness to marry. This bride wears her marriage jewelry.* right *In Arnhem Land, boys are circumcised as part of their initiation rites, when they are between the ages of eight and ten. Once the initiate has been*

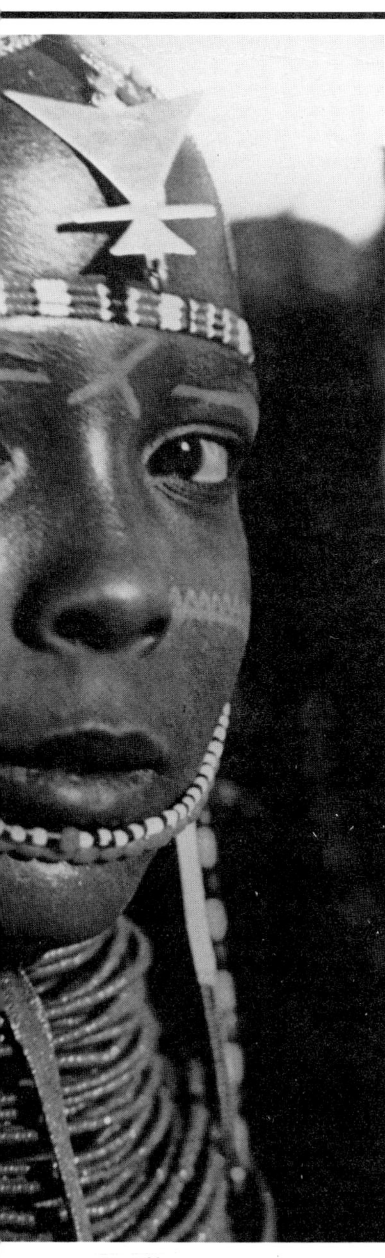

*prepared by painting, special relatives bear him to the ceremonial ground for the final ritual.*

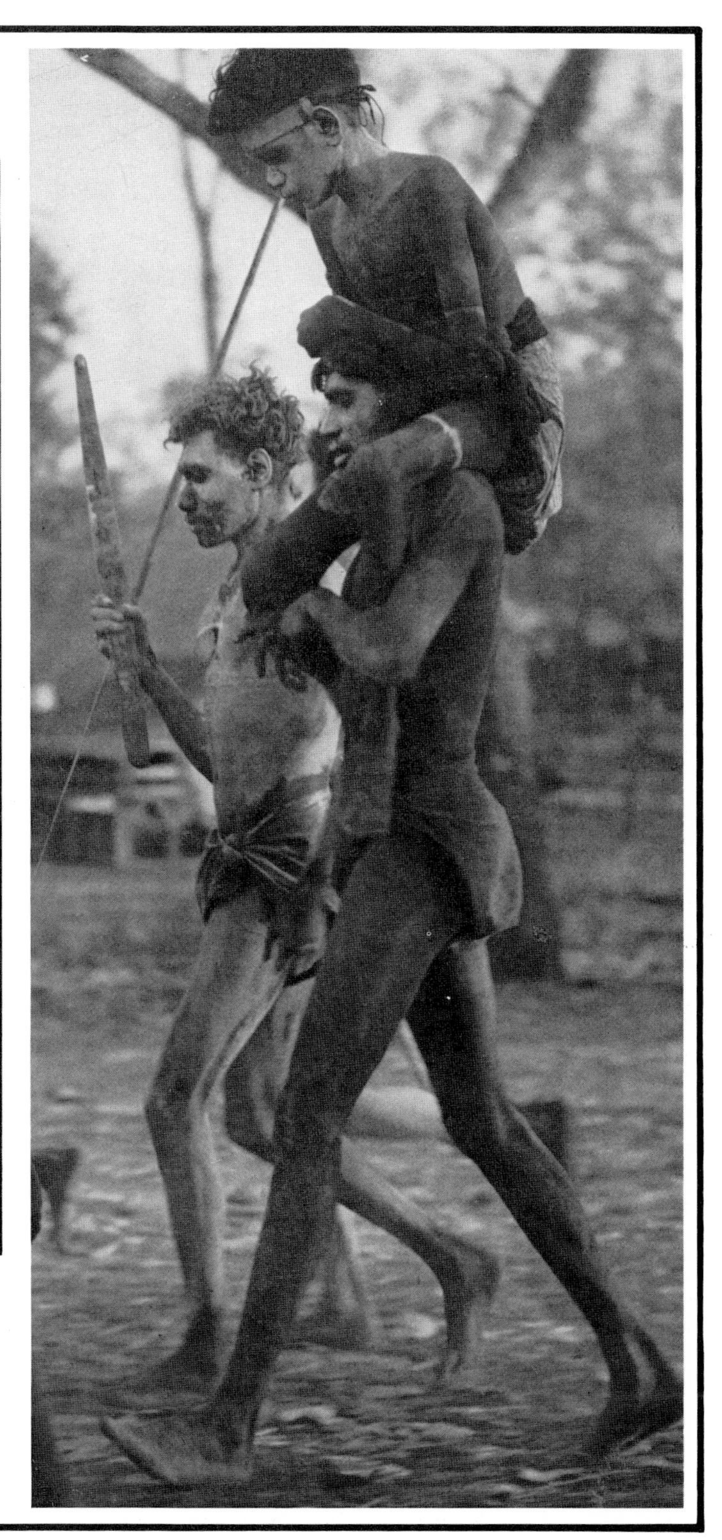

members of the community as an adult woman. (On Melville Island, off Darwin, the girl is painted red and yellow by the father, who also dresses her hair, building it up into a mop by twisting the curled strands of human hair on top of a bamboo chaplet, attached to which is an ornament of flattened dogs' tails set in beeswax.)

Marriage for the Australian woman may occur before or after this ceremony. Before they marry, although there is no true female circumcision in Australia, the girls undergo a physical operation, which in north-western Queensland took the form of introcision of the vagina. This was performed on the brides and the posterior vaginal margin, known as the fourchette, was torn and the hymen artificially ruptured.

The great Australian initiation rites involve the circumcision and subincision of young men. Prior to this, the first operation involving body alteration is the piercing of the nasal septum, a rite that seems to have little more symbolic significance than ear-piercing for us. The next operation, carried out on both boys and girls, usually at puberty, is tooth excision, when one or two of the front teeth are removed. The means is simple and the ritual minimal. The child is taken to a special spot by his cousin (normally a mother's brother's son), told to lie on his back, and held tightly while the operator carefully strips back the gum from around the tooth with a sharp, pointed stick. The stick is pressed against the tooth and hit with a stone until the tooth is loose enough to be removed with the fingers and held up in triumph for all to see.

The initiation involving circumcision, subincision and scarification takes place after puberty. During the circumcision and the accompanying ceremonies the boys are painted white. At the end of their seclusion, they wash off the paint and anoint themselves with fat. Their re-entry into society as adults is celebrated by painting them with red ochre. Circumcision was traditionally performed with a sharp stone, although they now use the safety razor-blade. This mutilation of the body symbolizes the rebirth of the initiate into a new world of adult men, a world of secrets hidden from women and children. He learns some of the sacred story of creation and begins to play his own role in the ceremonies of the tribe. Subincision, the splitting open of the urethra, takes place later still. This is another status symbol, for within the tribes where it is practised, a man cannot marry or enter the higher mysteries until the operation has been performed.

The final passage rite is death, when the corpse and the

mourners are decorated in honour of the occasion. Widows and other mourners are covered with ashes or white pipe clay; during this time the widows are forbidden to speak. For a young child, a mother may chop off a finger joint; for a husband, the women wail and mutilate their scalps with their digging sticks. After a woman has completed her time of seclusion and silence and is ready to re-marry, she removes her mourning paint and paints herself with red and yellow ochre and sometimes charcoal. She applies these colours in vertical bands or lines over the chest and back and in horizontal lines across the shoulders.

A few hours after death, among the Murngin, the relatives who belong to the dead man's clan, led by the father if he is alive, paint the design of his clan upon him. The paintings and designs are exactly the same as those placed on the young boy when he is circumcised and when he first saw the sacred totemic paraphernalia. First, the body is smeared with grease and painted all over with red ochre. The totemic designs are painted on the chest and abdomen; the hair is cut or plucked out to make into a sacred hair belt, and the scalp is painted white. The painting is done so that the ancestors can see the totem the man belonged to and carry the soul immediately to its proper resting place, just as the Sioux tattoos acted as a passport to the land of the ghosts.

A considerable amount of pain is inevitable during the mutilations which take place at various Australian passage rites and it has been suggested that this element of pain is an essential part of the marking of the body during this most critical passage rite. As the boys are changed into men, and the girls into women, they become permanently and painfully aware of their new role.

This can be well demonstrated among the Samoans, if one accepts the anthropologist G. B. Milner's explanation. Samoan men, instead of being circumcised and subincised, were tattooed at puberty and in early manhood. Considerable areas of the body from the waist to the knees, including the thighs, were covered with intricate geometrical designs, portions of which were completely covered with pigment. It was a lengthy business and very painful. There was always extensive bleeding and this was sometimes attended by septicaemia and death. During the tattooing, which was performed by a specialist and his assistant, the patient's courage was kept up by pretty girls who sang and cosseted him. The completed design was hidden away, only small portions of the tattoo at the knees and waist being visible under the sarong. Milner suggests that this tattooing was similar to an initiation rite, rather than being created for aesthetically pleasing and sexually exciting reasons. The boy became a man. More precisely, the function of the tattooing was rather like the couvade ceremony when the father takes himself to bed and receives the congratulations of friends and kin. Since a Samoan woman, to become fully adult, must undergo the painful initiation of bearing her first child, a man redressed the balance of the sexes by undergoing tattooing, whereby through an ordeal of blood and pain he became an adult in a way analogous to the child-bearing woman. Men's tattooing gave pain to them and joy to the women who glimpsed the artwork; childbirth gave pain to women and joy to the men who became fathers.

If we can try to understand passage rites and the body decoration that accompanies them as ceremonies which both imprint a new status on the individual and at the same time serve to introduce him by degrees into the mysteries of the social organization of a group, then we are likely to appreciate a truer picture.

# Conclusion

LIKE MOST BOOKS, *The Decorated Body* has been divided into a number of chapters dealing with separate themes. In this way I have somewhat artificially stressed certain aspects of body art, isolating the 'religious', 'symbolic' and 'social', for instance, for the sake of anthropological argument. In fact, the subject cannot be neatly split up into themes. The meanings of body decoration are too complex, and superficially similar methods have diverse ends. Thus, Maori *moko* tattooing expresses the status of a wealthy and admired warrior, whereas the haphazard tattooing of a Borstal boy symbolizes membership of a group; Ibo facial scarification indicates tribal identity, while German duelling scars are signs of virility; Hindus paint their faces as a mark of ritual purity, and Western women powder their noses to gain self-confidence or an impression of youthfulness.

Body decoration in some societies is the most important of the arts, and in many cases may justly be termed a fine art. However, for myself as an anthropologist, the most interesting fact to have emerged from researching and writing this book is that the transformation through art of the human body is a basic need which is universally practised among the peoples of the world, even the most puritanical or the most simple. In all societies the man or woman who is not decorated—in some way changed from their natural animal state—is, in a sense, dumb. Like body gesture, body decoration is a kind of language or code which is spoken through hairstyles, mutilation, tattooing or painting.

In the West, with our obsession with clothing for almost all parts of our body, from ear-muffs to socks and shoes, we have restricted the amount of skin available to be used as a cosmetic language. Most of us have forgotten that perhaps the first works of art dedicated to the combination of form and colour were carried out on the skin. Clothing has worked to the detriment of our appreciation of the human body painted or scarred into a harmonious work of art. Our code, dominated by fashion, is based on our 'second skin', our clothes.

Nevertheless, there are signs that the body is coming into its own again, with a more adventurous use of body paint and a sort of renaissance of the more permanent body arts. We are beginning to realize that we can express ourselves through painting, which is of course an ephemeral art and can be washed off after the performance, the party or when a special situation changes. The tattoos and scars of the Punk movement, of adolescents and gangs, remain on the skin-canvas as long as the subject lives, and even longer.

In a world becoming grey with fog and cement and conformity, an adventurous approach to our bodies may provide us with a welcome sense of personal freedom, of creative impulse. For example, although cosmetics are dominated by fashion, they may provide a woman with the chance to reveal her inner feelings. We should attempt to come to terms again with our bodies, using them for genuine aesthetic purposes in the same way as the Australians and Polynesians do when they paint for dances and tattoo for beauty. Perhaps if we came to terms with our skins as canvas, we might be able to relate to our physical being in a saner way, and overcome the need for freakish expressions of inner confusion such as orgiastic meals, exaggerated sexual contact or the even more absurd manipulation of the bodies of our pets and even our cars.

Attention to the body is an attempt to put on a new skin, a cultural as opposed to a natural skin. African hunters may paint to protect their bodies from the sun, the wind or insects, in the same way as we clothe ourselves for practical purposes. However, their main aim is no more 'practical' than our reasons for choosing the clothes we wear—nor is it out of modesty. No naked primitive paints to cover his nakedness, but he may paint his face to protect himself from the tangible and intangible forces of the forest, just as an American or European woman wears a slash of red on her lips to protect herself from the tangible and intangible forces of the suburbs, and feels 'naked' without it. It is a basic need. Even during famines, Kalahari Bushmen continue to smear their wives with animal fat, though food is desperately short; and during recent world wars, cosmetics were made available on almost the same terms as meat, butter, sugar and tea, in recognition of their importance in maintaining the morale of a fighting nation.

Cosmetics help an individual's appearance, and as Tolstoy wrote in *Childhood*, 'nothing has so marked an influence on the direction of a man's mind as his appearance, and not his appearance itself, so much as his conviction that it is attractive or unattractive.' This is how we should understand the satisfaction of a man smeared with soot and ochre in the New

Guinea mountains or of a woman smeared with soot and ochre in a Miami bar. This is how we should understand the Tasmanian woman observed by Peron in the eighteenth century:

> Ourê-Ourê showed us for the first time the kind of paint in these regions, and the manner of its application. Having taken some charcoal in her hands, she reduced it to a very fine powder; then putting it in her left hand, she took some in her right, rubbed first of all her forehead, and then both her cheeks and in a moment made herself black enough to frighten one; what seemed to us most singular was the complacency with which this young girl appeared to regard us after this operation and the confident air which this new ornament had spread over her physiognomy. (Quoted from Ling Roth)

Cosmetics, therefore, may do wonders for morale and self-confidence. Today, doctors are sending hypochondriacs and genuine invalids to beauty resorts as part of their general medical therapy, and cosmetic surgery is increasingly being considered by health services as necessary psychiatric and psychotherapeutic treatment. Cosmetics, therefore, *pace* some sociologists, should not be seen as manipulations of innocent people, but rather a way of liberating them. Instead of attacking the painted lady, feminists should encourage the gentlemen to paint.

The matter goes even deeper. Body painting, tattooing, even hairstyles, are concerned with the perennial questions all human beings have asked: 'Who am I? Who are we?' As long as there is an attempt to find an answer, people will continue to make up. A sane perception of self is closely linked with a sane perception of the body. As we paint our eyes, trim our body hair, put on our ties, belts and ribbons, we are creating a self-portrait of ourselves. Both the American typist and the Polynesian warrior are telling other people through signs that they are special kinds of individuals.

If we realize the importance of bodily transformation, we may have a better understanding of the American-inspired 'beauty culture'. We are arriving at a point where appearance is becoming everything. While much of this book has been about the devotion of so-called primitive peoples to caring for their body image, members of this new beauty culture may be said to be wallowing in its pursuit. Even men, proudly declaring their indifference to personal vanity, spend hours every day in mirrored bathrooms, conditioning their hair, their skin and their nails. The modern beauty imperative is becoming an obsessional time- and money-consuming ordeal. We fight fat, build muscles, wear hairpieces and sit under sun-ray lamps in a frenzy to keep up the appearance of wealth or health or youth. Our daughters start early with make-up kits for the twelve-year-old; and our wives have facials and a hairdo as others have a fix—in order to forget their frustrations and tensions. As when entering the drugged or drunken state for a short time, they are irresponsibly safe.

At their worst, Western beauty rites have become an indulgence, a way of filling in time or propping up disintegrating personalities, concealing not only lines and wrinkles but inner distress. Hopeless people are given something to believe in, and they can challenge the inevitability of death through a mask of paint. Yet this use of cosmetics is very different from the expressive painting and marking of the body described throughout this book. We have become deaf to the meaning of the body in association with art. Like us, the Polynesians and Amerindians had their 'beauty cultures', their saunas or sweat baths, and their vanity bags. Polynesians anointed their skin with scents and oils as well as tattooing it; they also blanched it by keeping brides and princesses under cover for long months.

However, the purpose of the primitive beautician was much more than putting on a mask. In figuring or colouring the skin they aimed to imprint on the mind all the traditions and philosophy of a group; the body was used to convey messages about the values held in common. Body art was basic to primitive man's social and aesthetic outlook and to his relationship with the natural and the supernatural world.

Perhaps we shall never again learn to paint and thereby communicate with our bodies. The world is running away with us, and we are faced with such a momentum of social change that our minds—much more than our bodies—are not able to keep up with it. For a harmonious fusion of society, beliefs and the decorated body, we need stable, homogeneous groups. Tattooing, scarification and painting as art forms belong to the lost world of the primitive. It seems that, after all, our own world is condemned to mass-produced cosmetics, wigs and other beauty aids, and that our body decoration will never again be dictated to by social needs, aesthetic ideals or religious beliefs, but by Fashion.

# Reading List

Barton, F. R. 1918 'Tattooing in South-Eastern New Guinea' *Journal of the Royal Anthropological Institute*

Becher, H. 1973 'Die Haartracht der Yanomami Indianer Nordwest Braziliens als Ausdrucksmittel religioser Vorstellung' *Kosmetologie*

Bohannan, Paul 1956 'Beauty and Scarification among the Tiv' *Man*

Brain, Robert & Pollock, Adam 1971 *Bangwa Funerary Sculpture* London

Brain, Robert 1976 *Friends and Lovers* London

Darwin, Charles 1890 *Journals and Researches . . . During the Voyage in H.M.S. Beagle* London

Dingwall, Eric John 1931 *Artificial Cranial Deformation*

Faris, James C. 1972 *Nuba Personal Art* London

Genet, Jean 1966 *Our Lady of the Flowers* London

Hallpike, C. R. 1969 'Social Hair' *Man* NS4

Hambly, W. D. 1925 *The History of Tattooing and its Significance* London

Hansen, H. H. 1972 'Clitoridectomy: female circumcision in Egypt' *Folk*

Karsten, Sigfrid Rafael 1926 *The Civilisation of South American Indians*

Kupka, Karel 1972 *Peintures aborigines d'Australie* Paris

Leach, E. R. 1958 'Magical Hair' *Journal of the Royal Anthropological Institute*

Lebeuf, Jean-Paul 1953 'Labrets et greniers des Falis' *Bulletin de l'Institut françois d'Afrique*

Levi-Strauss, Claude 1961 *Tristes Tropiques* New York
1968 'The Art of Asia and America' *Structural Anthropology* London

Lincoln, Bruce 1975 'The religious significance of women's scarification among the Tiv' *Africa* vol. 45

Ling Roth, H. *The Aborigines of Tasmania*

McGregor, Frances Cooke 1974 *Transformation and Identity* The Hague

Melville, Herman 1958 *Typee* London

Milner, G. B. 1969 'Siamese twins and the double helix' *Man* NS4

Munn, Nancy D. 1973 *Walbiri Iconography* London

Paulme, Denise 1973 'Adornment and Nudity in Tropical Africa' *Primitive Art and Society* (ed. Forge, Anthony) Oxford

Perutz, Kathrin 1972 *Beyond the Looking Glass: Life in the Beauty Culture* London

Plath, Sylvia 1969 'The fifteen-dollar eagle' *Penguin Modern Stories 2* London

Polhemus, Ted & Procter, Lynn 1978 *Fashion and Anti-fashion* London

Richie, D. 1974 'Japanese Tattooing' *Natural History* 10
Robley, H. G. 1896 *Moko or Maori Tattooing* London

Seeger, Anthony 1975 'The Meaning of Body Ornaments' *Ethnology* July
Skutt, Ronald & Gotch, Christopher 1974 *Skin Deep: The Mystery of Tattooing* London
Steinen, Karl von den 1925 *Die Marquesaner und ihre Kunst* Berlin
Strathern, Andrew and Marilyn 1971 *Self-decoration in Mount Hagen* London

Teit, James A. 1927–8 'Tattooing and Face- and Body-painting of Thompson Indians of British Columbia' *45th Annual Report of the Ethnological Bureau* Washington
Turner, V. 1966 'Colour classification in Ndembu ritual in Banton' *Anthropological Approaches to the Study of Religion* (ed. Michael)

Zahan, Dominique 1975 'Colours and body painting in Black Africa: the problem of the "half-man"' *Diogenes* Spring Paris

# Index

*Page references to illustrations are printed in italic and refer to the pages on which the captions are printed.*